AUG 2008 WF

FO **SALMONELLA**

Food, sex, and salmonella Why our food is ma
615.9 WALTNER

39204000024415

223449

DATE DUE

APR 2 9 2010	

DEMCO, INC. 38-2931

Dr. DAVID WALTNER-TOEWS

FOOD, SEX, AND SALMONELLA

WHY OUR FOOD IS MAKING US SICK

GREYSTONE BOOKS
Douglas & McIntyre Publishing Group
Vancouver/Toronto/Berkeley

Greystone Books
A division of Douglas & McIntyre Ltd.
2323 Quebec Street, Suite 201
Vancouver, British Columbia
Canada V5T 4S7
www.greystonebooks.com

Library and Archives Canada Cataloguing in Publication
Waltner-Toews, David, 1948–
Food, sex and salmonella : why our food is making us sick / David Waltner-Toews.

Includes index.
ISBN 978-1-55365-271-7

1. Foodborne diseases. 2. Foodborne diseases—Prevention. 1. Title.
RA601.5.W34 2008   615.9'54   C2007-905228-2

Editing by Nancy Flight
Copy editing by Viola Funk
Cover design by Peter Cocking
Text design by Jessica Sullivan
Printed and bound in Canada by Friesens
Printed on acid-free paper that is forest friendly (100% post-consumer
recycled paper) and has been processed chlorine free.
Distributed in the U.S. by Publishers Group West

We gratefully acknowledge the financial support of the Canada Council for the
Arts, the British Columbia Arts Council, the Province of British Columbia through
the Book Publishing Tax Credit, and the Government of Canada through the Book
Publishing Industry Development Program (BPIDP) for our publishing activities.

This book is dedicated to
my partners in foodborne disease crime over
the past couple of decades, especially
Scott McEwen, Linda Harris, Andria Jones,
Dominique Charron, and Sandy Lefebvre.

Nothing is so much to be shunned as sex relations.
All diseases of Christians are to be ascribed to demons.
Give me chastity and continence, but not yet.
ST. AUGUSTINE (from various writings)

CONTENTS

PREFACE TO THE SECOND EDITION

THIS BOOK IS ABOUT LOVE, EATING, AND GETTING SICK.

AT LEAST one reviewer of this book's first edition complained that she couldn't find the sex and felt misled. She had, I think, quite a narrow view of love, of eating, and of sex. Others wondered if the title was *Food, Sex, and Salmonella,* or *Food Sex and Salmonella,* the latter apparently having somewhat risqué overtones. The first chapter explains all that, so I won't spend valuable words expounding my theories here. Still, I did return to the literature and discovered that some foodborne diseases can be sexually transmitted. You will need to do a bit of work—to read the book—to find them. I hope that you will find this work pleasurable. Easy food, like easy sex, leads us down a path to waste and destruction of ourselves and the planet we live on. I have tried to make this book inviting but not too easy.

There are many hazards in the kitchen, including the hot, spraying fat, the risk of being burned to death as an unwanted wife in some parts of India, and, in the last few years in North America, a new phenomenon. A letter in the 1991 issue of the *New England Journal of Medicine* told the story of a healthy teenager who heated seven intact eggs in the microwave. As he removed them from the microwave and sat down at the table, six of the eggs exploded simultaneously, spraying him across the face; he suffered second-degree burns across his eyes, nose, and forehead. This book is not about that kind of hazard. It's about infection and disease.

The danger of writing a book like this is that I will overwhelm you with facts about bacteria, viruses, and parasites and endless lists of foodborne disease outbreaks and cases. The facts are all very well and good, but unless someone makes sense of them, they are not of much use. The way scientists make sense of facts is by telling convincing stories. All the models and statistics and experimentally derived facts are ways of corroborating stories (or not). And the stories are never just about what scientists think.

Because foodborne diseases are of great, global, public health importance, everybody should be able to engage in lively, knowledgeable conversation about them so that we can have better-run restaurants, farms, kitchens, farmers' markets, greengrocers, and butcher shops. We should all be telling stories about foodborne diseases, making jokes about them, and creating excellent public policies and programs to contain them or to live with them. Every story tells something about the storyteller. I was recently mocked by a business reporter for suggesting that ecomonies of scale, such as those espoused by Wal-Mart, were in some way responsible for pandemics of salmonellosis and avian flu. To me, his mocking suggested a profound ignorance of both biology and global trade. He might agree with storytellers who suggest that the problems of foodborne diseases can be easily solved if people was their hands and cook their food and that the increasing flows and changing patterns of bacteria and viruses around the globe are irrelevant (or uncontrollable).

As will become clear as you read this book, I believe that personal behavior is important but that this behavior is embedded in changing social, economic, and ecological patterns around the world. Hand washing and global warming and economies of scale are all important contributors to the changing nature of pandemics. We need all the evidence we can dig up and all the stories we can tell to make sense of that evidence.

In the course on foodborne diseases that I have been teaching for twenty years, I have students prepare what I call a dissemination project. They pick a group of people they think needs to know something about a particular foodborne illness or group of illnesses. Then they create an appropriate way to communicate with that group. Some of them come up with the usual sermons or tracts and posters that are the hallmark of much (really bad) public health communication. But over the years, they have also given me videos ("The Young and the Retching" comes to mind), educational dinners at synagogues and churches, websites, booklets for students and hitchhikers, and songs for the radio, day-care center, or campfire.

This book, like those dissemination projects, is less about the diseases themselves than about who gets them and why, what messages they are sending to us from the natural world of which we are a part, and how we can take pressure off the disease care system and create a more convivial world through how we eat.

Some basic material about foodborne diseases hasn't changed much since 1992, when the first edition of this book was published. Our understanding about the way the human body gets sick, for instance, is pretty much the same now as it was twenty years ago, and several of the diseases, like botulism and salmonellosis, have been around so long that they almost seem "normal." As Canadian singer Bruce Cockburn said, "The trouble with normal is it always gets worse." Indeed, what we consider normal has changed; we no longer talk about eradicating salmonellosis, as some people used to, and botulism has re-established itself as a major disease in several countries of the former Soviet Union, giving people a deadly taste of what happens when we don't invest in public health infrastructure or aggressively regulate private industry.

But the kinds of outbreaks and epidemics we see today are different from what they were twenty years ago. They are often bigger, usually more geographically dispersed, always more difficult to investigate. It is no great comfort to me that I said this would happen, and my critics scoffed, in the early 1990s.

Some new diseases have become discernible from the background noise in the last couple of decades. These are called "emerging diseases," and there are whole journals devoted to them. The assessment of the burden imposed on society by foodborne illnesses has also changed; it's worse than we thought. But there is also a convergence of understanding as to how we might begin to think about, and respond to, the whole complex interacting mess of eating, agriculture, urbanization, economics, and epidemics of foodborne diseases.

Well, the convergence is emerging among people who agree with me. But that is a whole lot more people now than it was two decades ago. You might even be one of them. You won't know until you read this book, will you? Think of this book as my dissemination project. When you are finished reading, go to my website, send me an e-mail, and give me a grade. Then vote for a better world with your feet, your hands, and your menu for the week.

A word about the organization of this book. The chapters in the first section ("French Kissing on the First Date") are an introduction to the personal and global dimensions of foodborne diseases. They give new reasons to think about food and sex and describe in some nauseating detail how food can make a person sick.

The second section of the book ("When She Stays for Breakfast") deals with problems in food associated with bacteria, bacterial toxins, viruses, and parasites. This section begins with chapters on foodborne and waterborne infections (which usually show up in people primarily as diarrhea); these are followed by two chapters on intoxications by bacterial products, one focusing on the "usual" intoxications, in which vomiting is usually the prominent sign, and one on botulism, which has its own unique history and clinical signs and symptoms. This section concludes with rollicking, gut-wrenching, mind-bending tales of parasites and a variety of natural poisons found in seafood.

The third section of the book ("When She Moves In") tackles all those things that we don't normally connect with vomiting and diarrhea but that worry us because they may cause long-term problems—things like chemicals, antibiotics, and poisons produced by molds. Finally, the last section ("Spicing Up the Long-Term Commitment") comes back to how we can think about all these complicated problems and what kinds of solutions are available to us.

At the end, if you really want to know more, and the rack next to the toilet is in need of something besides collections of wit and wisdom, I have suggested some further readings.

PREFACE
TO THE
FIRST
EDITION

THIS IS NOT another book to tell you that your food is saturated with poisons and that you need a special guidebook if you want to survive. Nor will I tell you that the food you eat is the safest in the world and that you need not worry because General Foods will take care of you. Nor will I exhort you to fill up on oat bran and lettuce to avert a heart attack or to eat more beef to help save the farmers. Increasingly, the acts of everyday life, eating, and the transfiguration of food into flesh and fertilizer, appear to involve agonizing, globally significant choices, explained to us by self-important authors in technical tomes and prophetic warnings.

Eating does involve globally significant choices, and this book will explain what they are. But, as Beatle George Harrison once said, life goes on within you and without you. In the end, this is a book about enjoying—no, thrilling at—the true meaning of eating. It is about intimacy, love, vomiting, and diarrhea. This book is about the celebration of ecology through eating and about how foodborne disease can save the world.

This book should be kept next to your toilet and also next to the refrigerator. The next time you are doubled over with abdominal pain, feeling like you have never felt before the true revolution within, feeling like your liver is coming up your throat, like you want to die, I want you to understand what is happening to you, why the inner child is having a gaseous tantrum in your guts. I want you to hear Gaia's, the earth organism's, whispered love message to you so that your suffering is not in vain. I want you to feel good about yourself, to return to the table with fire in your eyes, laughter in your belly, and hands that have been very thoroughly washed.

This is your mother talking. Did you remember to flush? Read on.

FRENCH KISSING
ON THE
FIRST DATE

FOOD, SEX, AND SALMONELLA

WHAT'S THE
PROBLEM?

A ONE-YEAR-OLD child will put anything into her mouth, just to taste what it is. As we get older, we get more squeamish and more sophisticated; we say, "Let me see what you've got," not "Let me taste what you've got." But we do continue to stick strange and wonderful things into our mouths and to stick our tongues into, and around in, amazing places, well into adulthood. We call it eating. And the more socially unacceptable our chosen food, the more apt we are to call it gourmet food or health food or an acquired taste, as if its acquisition implied a higher plane of evolution.

Eating is one of the great sensual pleasures of life. It is where that fuzzy sense of mystical at-oneness with the world meets, and celebrates hard biological necessity. When we eat we are, quite literally, turning the world outside in. Foods are nothing more or less than pieces of environments: bark, leaves, roots, sap of trees (maple syrup, date palm juice), and animals of all sorts from the land and the sea, even bacteria (think live-culture yogurt), algae. We even eat dirt. I have a report in my files of a woman who habitually ate earth, with its associated beetles and the like, from the graves of priests. She subsequently suffered infection with the cat roundworm *Toxocara cati.*

Most of us do not eat dirt in that way, of course, although pica (abnormal appetites), which includes the eating of dirt, is more common than we realize. Ever watch a one-year-old child in the sandbox? But even adults are not immune to such behavior, and normality, particularly with regard to food preferences, is very much culturally conditioned. In the end, eating dirt in some African cultures is really no different from eating mineral supplements in North America.

When we eat, we select portions of an environment and bring them into intimate contact with our bodies. They become one with us, and we become one with the earth. What sex is to interpersonal relationships, eating is to the human-environment relationship, a daily consummation of our marriage to the living biosphere.

We have been having this intimate relationship with the planet, sticking our tongues into new and exciting environments, since before we became human, since, as it were, our very first date.

And, like sexual promiscuity and ignorance of our sexual partners, promiscuity in eating habits and ignorance of eating "partners" can carry great risks. When we eat or drink indiscriminately, who knows what a circus of viruses, parasites, and bacteria we are ingesting?

Among the animals of earth, none are more promiscuous, none more deserving of the adjective "omnivorous," than people.

Eating is one of those wonderfully ambiguous activities that put us both a little lower than the angels and a (very) little higher than the dust from which we are made.

North Americans, as well as Australians, New Zealanders, and Europeans, are displaced persons from every continent on earth. Given that eating is such an intimate relationship with the environment, it should not be surprising that we have carried our eating preferences with us to these new lands. It would seem fickle not to do so. As a result, North Americans from rice cultures continue to follow a rice-based diet, immigrants from the Ukraine still want cabbage borscht like Oma made, and those from the Caribbean long for succulent kingfish. Some items, like cabbage, may be grown in our new homes. Others cannot and hence must be imported from environments thousands of miles away.

Although global trade in food products is probably less than 20 percent of total world production, its economic value has increased more than tenfold since the 1960s, and the environmental and public health impacts of these traded foods are huge. The international food trade has greatly influenced our perception of food, the shape of the food industry, and the kinds of food safety issues that plague us. Eating has become for some people a form of nostalgia for another time, another place, and another season, even as, for others, it is an act of adventure and rebellion. These are pretty heavy burdens for carrots, hamburgers, cabbage, and chicken to be carrying around.

When I talk to people about food safety issues and suggest that maybe we should look at alternative ways of producing and distributing food, I sense a deep anxiety, bordering on paranoia, in many of the responses I get. Many in the modern food industries see moves to constrain the distribution of food as veiled attempts to plunge us back into the dark, cold, hungry days of the Middle Ages. They wax sentimental about the simpler days of the 1970s, when intensification of food production and mass distribution were seen simply as effective business responses to a combination of hunger, nostalgia, rebellion, and population growth.

Trade in human foods and animal feeds amounting to billions of dollars annually supports this hunger, nostalgia, and adventurism. Shipping of foods over long distances can cause serious problems of spoilage. Nevertheless, developments in preservation technology since the late nineteenth century, especially refrigeration, have allowed international trade in perishable items such as meat and fish to flourish. It is instructive to look at the food trade figures for Europe and North America, not as an accountant or a financial bookkeeper might, but from an ecologist's point of view. We trade in fresh, chilled, and frozen meat, dairy products, eggs, honey, fruits, vegetables, and grains with hundreds of countries around the world. North American eaters, who are typical of those in most industrialized countries, are physically married to environments from Burundi to Belize, from New Caledonia to the Netherlands. Globally, this state is not unusual.

In the early years of this millennium, Lisa Deutsch and her colleagues in the Department of Systems Ecology at Stockholm University tried to trace the origins of Swedish foods. They found this task challenging, since foods at point of consumption are not always labeled according to where they came from but rather according to where they were "made"—that is, packaged or reformulated. They found that ecosystems from Southeast Asia, South America, and continental Europe subsidized a large proportion of what the public thought was a sustainable "made in Sweden" agriculture. About 80 percent of manufactured animal feeds for pigs, chickens, and cattle, for instance, depended on imported ingredients. Consumers who are checking out the farms in their own countryside often pay attention to the wrong things; the environmental damage and the trade in bacteria, viruses, and parasites are well out of view. The *Salmonella* are stowaways on ships and airplanes crisscrossing the globe, feeding the industrialized countries' frenzy for all the food, all the time. Out of sight, out of mind.

On top of this, more people are traveling than ever before in history, either as economic, environmental, or political refugees or as free-wheeling tourists. International migrants increased from 75 million in 1960 to more than 190 million in 2005, almost 3 percent of the world's population. International tourist arrivals—the number of tourists arriving at their destinations—increased from about 25 million to 650 million between 1950 and 1999. If the foods cannot come to us, we are going to them.

Not only separated from our ancestral homes, we are increasingly displaced from a rural to an urban environment. Since 1950, the proportion of people living in cities has almost doubled; in 2005, almost half of all people lived in urban areas. By 2030, that proportion will be 60 percent. The students in my class on foodborne diseases, taught at a university that prides itself on its agricultural origins, are typical of students just about everywhere in the world. They have never been on farms. They have no real idea where food comes from. They are thus estranged even from those foods that can be grown nearby. This double displacement means that most of us are, in effect, carrying on intimate relationships with environments of which we have no knowledge; it is like engaging in sex with a blindfold on. Just as reducing individuals with personalities and histories to anonymous sexual objects defined only by physical characteristics can lead to abusive relationships with people, so reducing foods from biological entities with specific ecological histories to tradable commodities defined by price, fiber, fat, or protein content has resulted in an abusive relationship with the environment.

We now have urban economists and developers who can without embarrassment talk about the loss of farmland to urbanization as progress or necessity, or as a matter of esthetic choices, jobs versus environment, or some other nonsensical juxtaposition of options. They can naively speak of food as if it were a simple commodity, like shoes or condoms. I have heard suggestions that agriculture is a tiny part of the national economy and therefore, by implication, unimportant. Under which stones do they find these policymakers and economists? I suggest that they be forced to do without the products of agriculture as they reconsider the importance of agriculture. Maybe a light bulb would go on somewhere. Do you mean food comes from farms?

We even have public health advocates fighting diseases such as avian influenza by promoting economies of scale and high biosecurity (putting all your eggs in one basket and guarding it well) when all the evidence says that every basket, sooner or later, gets dropped. The result of this ignorance will surely be a continued loss of farmland, the loss of the biological food-producing foundation of our civilization, and the degradation of rural environments. It will mean increased intensity and scale in food production and in processing and distribution systems, increased abuse of farm animals, increased levels (because of increased stress-related shedding and increased cross-contamination) and distribution (because of centralization and economies of scale) of foodborne pathogens, increased use of chemicals or high-energy technology to control those pathogens (in response to urban demands), and the undermining of the ability of both farmers and consumers to make free and intelligent decisions about their food.

What may save us yet—and it may sound perverse for me to wish this—are the foodborne illnesses that follow us around the world and from the countryside to the city. For microbes and parasites, the invisible travelers through our kitchens, foods we eat are ecosystems unto themselves. Eating, from their viewpoint, is either just another way that humans plunder animals smaller than themselves or, just as often, a form of microbial self-perpetuation and extension into a new environment. In a real sense, we are simply an environment that allows bacteria, parasites, viruses, and chemicals to recycle themselves. The fact that they sometimes make us sick as they pass through is incidental and not to be confused with malicious intent.

These accidental infections are, alas, common. According to the World Health Organization, every year a billion people around the world get sick and about 2 million, mostly children under five years old, die because of infections transmitted to them in their food or water. The Centers for Disease Control and Prevention in the United States estimates that in the United States 76 million people a year get sick from foodborne diseases and five thousand people die from them. In the early 1980s, Ewen Todd of Health and Welfare Canada suggested that more than 2 million Canadians suffered from foodborne illnesses annually. More recent estimates put the number of foodborne illnesses in Canada at more than 11 million per year.

Nobody knows the real numbers. These estimates are just that. Estimating the magnitude of the risks of acute illness due to food is a bit of a casino game. Only a small fraction of cases—one in a few hundred for bacteria to one in thousands for viruses—ever gets counted. Not everyone with an intestinal problem visits the doctor. Even if one does suspect that the cause of one's illness is food, one may feel compelled to keep silent in the service of more lofty causes, such as the sanctity of Grandmother's cooking or a potential romantic liaison. The doctor may not do a sufficiently detailed workup to feel comfortable reporting your diarrhea as a case of foodborne disease. Not reporting it saves the doctor some paperwork. If there is a big outbreak following the supper at the church, mosque, temple, synagogue, or community hall, any individual doctor may treat only a few of the people that were affected and so may not be aware of the outbreak. If the doctor thought you were part of a bigger picture, he or she might report. The argument is cyclic; doctors do not report you because they do not know you are part of an epidemic, and they do not know you are part of an epidemic because all the other doctors are similarly ignorant.

Even if the doctor does report, the health agency may fail to conduct thorough investigations. First, for financially conservative governments, which consider public service a necessary evil at best, labor shortages and financial restrictions may be paramount. The government does not provide money or people to do these investigations unless there is a lot of public pressure. Second, local medical officers of health and health agencies may not want to look bad or stir up political trouble by reporting foodborne disease outbreaks. This may be not so much a conspiracy to cover up as a natural tendency not to want to throw indigestible items at a fan next to which one is sitting.

The estimates of millions of sick people from the World Health Organization, the Centers for Disease Control and Prevention, or the Public Health Agency of Canada may be accurate. True or not, these estimates are themselves used to estimate how many millions of dollars these diseases cost us as a society through lost income and productivity, loss of leisure time, suffering, and medical costs, as well as child-care costs while you were in bed, death (a minor item in this balance sheet), costs of recalling items and closing restaurants, and loss of international trade. Looked at in this light, a few trips to the toilet can take on cosmic significance. The assumption is that you would have been doing something productive had you gone to work. It overlooks the fact that the way our economy is set up, personal disaster is good for the gross national product. Consider, for instance, all those jobs created in the medical and insurance businesses, all on account of the custard on the counter you stuck your finger into. Personal catastrophe is good for the economy.

Several countries, as well as the World Health Organization, have instituted more active surveillance programs to try to get a clearer picture of what is going on, but overall measurement of the burden of disease from food is likely to remain a guessing game for some time to come. To a certain extent, doing the body counts of how many people get sick from food and water misses the point. We need to find ways to take better care of our food partners; they are the most important members of every economy on earth. We cannot live without food, so we are not in a great bargaining position. We need our food more than our food needs us; our relationship is not a one-night stand. Either we are in this for long-term commitment, or we can kiss the planet good-bye.

Although the exact number of people who get sick may be a good topic for a game of chance, every person who spends the night worshiping at the porcelain throne after the church picnic, every nursing home resident who dies from foodborne verotoxin-producing *Escherichia coli* (VTEC), and every woman who aborts from foodborne listeriosis makes a lie of the notion that we are free of the bounds of nature, that we can fornicate with the environment and not bear a cost.

In the long run, the risks associated with eating are considerably fewer than those associated with starvation. According to the Food and Agriculture Organization of the United Nations (FAO), there were more than 820 million undernourished people in the world in 2006. On the one hand, after some gains were made in improving the food supply in the 1970s and 1980s, the human race seems, at best, to be barely holding on. On the other, morally and physically gross, hand, in industrialized regions of the world, people are dying from eating too much; if I were in my (non–politically correct) veterinary frame of mind, I would say these people are fat and are dying from being fat, all the while complaining that the airplane seats are too small and the fast food has the wrong kinds of fat in it. The World Health Organization estimates that a billion adults worldwide are overweight and 300 million of them are clinically obese.

So all in all, the diseases described in this book are not catastrophic. Nevertheless, there are risks. In 2006, the week before my class lecture on *E. coli*, there was an outbreak of *E. coli* from spinach. The week before my lecture on botulism, half a dozen people were in hospitals across North America because they had chugged back all-natural carrot juice laced with all-natural botulism toxin. The week before my lecture on foodborne viruses, a couple of hundred students at a Canadian university ran for the stalls down the hall as part of an outbreak of Norwalk-like virus. My friends at the Public Health Agency of Canada were consulting my syllabus to see what illness they should prepare for next.

There is strong scientific evidence that the rates of foodborne disease in industrialized countries have been increasing as the result of global warming in the 1990s and into the twenty-first century; the patterns of those diseases have also been altered by trade, cultural, political, and environmental changes which I shall discuss in this book. The industrial methods developed to control foodborne diseases are, at best, pushing the rates down slightly for some diseases, but overall keeping them in a holding pattern. These diseases are not going away, and consumers (at last, a context in which it makes sense to describe people as consumers) should educate themselves about them, learn from them, and seek ways to reduce them. For me, the most convincing reason to pay attention to foodborne diseases is that they are part of our most intimate lifelong relationship. These diseases tell us as much about our complex relationships with the planet as STDs tell us about our contradictory relationships with each other. I have as much fun thinking about food as I do about sex. I hope you do as well.

This book is about understanding intimacy, about self-fulfillment, about you and your food partners. The next time you take a forkful of meat or rice or peas, ponder for a moment the environment with which you are about to become intimate. You may find that you wish to ask a few questions of it. You may want to know if she is a local girl, or if she just flew in from some exploited foreign environment. You may suddenly find yourself interested in the agricultural practices of Mexico, Spain, California, British Columbia, and Ontario. Good. This interest in your life's most intimate partner could be the start of something beautiful.

We may decide, like the good burghers of nineteenth-century Paris, that we do not wish to risk death for tasty bread. The following, quoted by noted microbiologist Theodor Rosebury in a wonderful, classic, must-read book, *Life on Man,* first appeared in "The Last Cholera Epidemic in Paris," in the *General Homeopathic Journal,* vol. 113, p. 15 (1886):

> The neighbours of the establishment famous for excellent bread, pastry, and similar products of luxury, complained again and again of the disgusting smells which prevailed therein and which penetrated into their dwellings. The appearance of cholera finally lent force to these complaints, and the sanitary inspectors who were sent to investigate the matter found that there was a connection between the water-closets of those dwellings and the reservoir containing water used in the preparation of the bread. The connection was cut off at once, but the immediate result thereof was a perceptible deterioration of the quality of the bread. Chemists have evidently no difficulty in demonstrating that water impregnated with "extract of water closet" has the peculiar property of causing dough to rise particularly fine, thereby imparting to bread the nice appearance and pleasant flavor which is the principal quality of luxurious bread.

Or we may, like many modern Japanese (and a few California chefs), decide that the risk of instant death that may come from an improperly cleaned puffer fish or the hole bored in one's stomach by *Anasakid* worms from parasitized salmon only adds spice to the delicate temptations of the flesh.

What is important is to know that we have choices, and that we own those choices, and to make them intelligently. The unexamined food, I would say, if I may be so bold as to take some license with Aristotle, is a risk not worth eating.

2

THE
VOICE OF
THE UNSEEN
GUEST

HOW PEOPLE

GET SICK

WHEN ANTON van Leeuwenhoek looked down his crude microscope in 1674 and discovered a world of "very little animalcules," he did not imagine that whole populations of these tiny creatures attended our every meal and entered our bodies unheralded. Or that there might be even smaller beasties, the viruses, inside the tiny bacteria he was seeing. Nor did those devout families who set out an extra chair for the Unseen Guest at their meals imagine that they were surrounded by millions of unseen guests who had no need of chairs.

Wading into the orgiastic world of microbes can be disconcerting. Why would any morally upright God create such an amoral mess of living things, breeding and crossbreeding, exchanging genetic material without regard for race, creed, species, or sexual preference? Right under our noses? Right *in* our noses? I am not a theologian, and cannot understand this, but we shall probably have to pinch our moral noses as we explore this world in order to rescue the maiden of our amazing and improbable lives.

When these microscopic bacteria and viruses enter our maws, riding on eggs and hamburgers as children in an amusement park might ride into a tunnel of ghosts, with what voices do they scream their joy and terror? How, in short, do they make us sick?

One might say that contaminants in our food can make us sick in one of two ways: through intoxication or through infection. Intoxications, caused by toxins in food, occur within minutes to hours after eating and are most often associated with vomiting. These are, technically, what we can call food poisoning. Infections, which require time for bacteria from the food to multiply inside the host's body before they cause havoc, develop hours and even days or weeks after eating, and the main sign is diarrhea. This would be called a foodborne infection. "Foodborne disease" covers both intoxications and infections.

Vomiting and diarrhea are the two most common characteristics of foodborne disease. I refer to them as "signs," which should be differentiated from "symptoms." Although many other writers are less careful in their use of these words than I am, the distinction is useful. A sign is what can be seen and measured in some way, like temperature, pulse, and the amount of water in your stool. A symptom is something you feel, like pain, a headache, or tingling in your fingertips. The distinction is obviously useful for a veterinarian, but it is also important for people. A doctor can (at least theoretically) measure a sign, even if the patient is a young child; you have to tell the physician about your symptoms. Most diseases present as a mixture of signs and symptoms.

If we call diarrhea a sign, which I would, you might well ask how we can measure it. Diarrhea occurs when a person's feces have increased water content above what we normally expect; not to put too fine a point on it, the feces flow, rather than plop. One could, of course, measure exact water content of a stool, but the simplest definition of diarrheic stool is that it takes the shape of the container into which it is put. Public health officials then usually say that a person has diarrhea if he or she has two or more (or occasionally three or more) such stools in a twenty-four-hour period.

Vomiting, also called emesis, occurs when your abdominal muscles and diaphragm contract, throwing the contents of the stomach and upper small intestine up through your esophagus and mouth (and, if you are really unlucky, your nose). Vomiting is controlled by a certain part of the brain, which is excited when it receives messages from certain nerves, many of which have endings in the stomach and upper small intestine. These nerve endings are switched on by both physical and chemical stimuli. As with diarrhea, the amount and timing of what comes out of your mouth could be measured, which is why I would call it a sign.

But there is more to this story than what comes out the orifices of one's body, instructive as that may be. Let us contemplate, for a moment, food as it passes our lips into the masticatory caverns where lurk the uncompromising teeth and the probing tongue. At the risk of self-absorbed intellectual implosion, let us further contemplate the tiny bacteria that may dwell within that food, whether they be friendly lactobacilli in yogurt, interloping *Salmonella* in cheese, or the parts per billion old or new chemicals that contaminate the interstices of complex carbohydrates or comprise the food itself. In so doing, you may gain some understanding of how you can get sick from so apparently a feeble sin as eating an egg soft boiled.

Forget, for a moment, the candle, the wine, that ambiguous look across the table. This is what it comes to: food is ground up and mixed with saliva in the mouth. Saliva contains, among other things, amylase, an enzyme to aid in digesting starch. It serves, as well, as a solvent for food chemicals, thus allowing one to taste them. Taste is a first defense against foodborne disease. I am quite suspicious of so-called acquired tastes. Not all foods that can make you sick taste bad, but—certain Danish cheeses, Chinese eggs, and Scandinavian putrefied fish aside— foul tastes and odors, metallic tastes, and burning sensations should serve as a warning.

Nevertheless, I confess that I, too, once polished off a bad-tasting steamed bun from a food court for a negligent nephew. It was from a Vietnamese fast food restaurant, and I felt a certain duty not only to eat the food but also to like it, as penance for coming from a culture that had behaved so miserably toward Vietnam. If I expected God to reward my virtue in finishing a bad-tasting bun, I was wrong. I not only felt miserable during the baked salmon candlelit dinner that evening but also spent what would have been the better part of my Christmas holidays bent over a porcelain throne, wishing I were dead. This kind of behavior may have something to do with parents who make an issue of food, drawing tight and judgmental arguments around the uneaten chicken and the starving children in India, China, or Ethiopia. Guilt and food are a common and deadly combination.

Our mouths have a large and complex natural bacterial flora that rarely cause any disease, unless you bite someone. Moreover, bacterial infections may put you off your food, but they seldom attack your mouth directly. Occasionally, foodborne diseases are associated with a sore throat. *Beta-hemolytic Streptococci,* the cause of strep throat, have managed on at least two occasions in the last decade to use food handlers to perpetuate themselves: once through a chocolate mousse fed to people at a blood bankers' conference in Kansas City and once through cold meatballs fed to soldiers at an Israeli military base.

Toxins—either those inherent in some foods, those added by our bacterial friends, or those that we add deliberately or inadvertently—are another matter. In very high doses they may induce irritation at the back of the pharynx, and hence retching, which is different from vomiting. Some toxins may produce burning or tingling sensations. What they do at low doses is the topic of a later chapter.

Safely past the teeth, the tongue, the tonsils, and the salivary glands, your food now takes that not-quite-irreversible plunge down the esophagus, white-water rafting on peristaltic waves down to your stomach. The image of a watery torrent is not so far off the mark. Consider for a moment the following estimated flow of fluids through your body every day: about 2 quarts of intake, 6 quarts of saliva and gastric, bile, and pancreatic juices, and 6 quarts of secretions from the intestines—for a total of 3 to 4 gallons! And these fluids are not just water; they contain all manner of essential electrolytes, such as sodium and potassium. Yet on a normal day in a normal person, less than a cup of that amount gets out the back door. Most of it is re-absorbed in the lower part of your intestines; this re-absorption is essential to maintain your body's fluid and electrolyte balance. It does not take much imagination to consider the havoc that might be wreaked by a small hole in the dike, the work of a tampering bacterium or virus.

At the stomach, the cardiac sphincter, the front door, opens to let food in but sometimes sprays a bit of acid up into the soft flesh of the esophagus, resulting in heartburn.

The stomach accepts the now somewhat sorry-looking foods as hand-me-downs from the mouth, grinds them into smaller particles, and churns up an emulsion of the fats. Sloshing about in this very acidic fluid, the food undergoes some preliminary digestion. As one might imagine, for the bacteria stowing away in our food, this acid bath is the most potentially deadly part of the ride.

If the collective bacterial mind thinks that our mouths provide easy access to the internal offices of the human body, they

are sadly mistaken. The lumen, or inside, of the gastrointestinal tract, from mouth to anus, is technically outside our bodies. While the inside of the gut has direct connections with the
world around you, and is full of all sorts of bacteria and viruses,
the true "inside" of your body is sterile. A heart surgeon has to
wear a mask and gloves to protect you from infection; my family
physician checking my prostate gland wears a glove to protect
her, not me. The gut is lined with protective barriers and guard-
ian cells. It is their job to let in only those molecules that know
the appropriate code words.

A great many bacteria die in the stomach. How, one might ask,
do any of them survive? Sometimes we unwittingly give them
help. An antacid taken for the heartburn, for instance, helps neu-
tralize the stomach's acids and makes it more comfortable not
just for you but for the little lives within you. Infants naturally
have less acidic stomach contents and so are more likely to give
the bacteria a home. Food may also protect the bacteria, which
snuggle unmolested in its depths. Furthermore, some vessels
give the bacteria a slower ride through the acid. Small amounts
of carbohydrates may pass through the stomach in thirty minutes or less. A high-fat meal may take several hours to move on.

With the exception of organisms such as *Helicobacter pylori,*
which causes ulcers and is probably transmitted through contaminated food and water, bacteria rarely find the stomach
sufficiently hospitable to take up residence there. Toxins are
a different matter. They may irritate the stomach directly or
may slip off to one's neural vomit center, where they stimulate a relaxation of the cardiac sphincter and esophagus, with
simultaneous contraction of the abdominal muscles and viscera.
Throwing up is an apt description; one might imagine a small
but powerful baseball player hiding in one's depths.

Toxins formed by the bacteria *Staphylococcus aureus* (which
hang around many people's noses) and *Bacillus cereus* (which
prefer rice fields) may attack in this way. Metals such as copper,

zinc, tin, and cadmium, if ingested in high doses, may do something similar. We might ingest such metals through leaching from a container or because our crops were grown in industrially contaminated soils.

Now that your food has survived a trip through the stomach, your gastronomic happiness rests in the hands of the small intestine, a 23-foot-long glistening, slithery tube. Although many toxins that can damage the stomach also attack this part of the gut, it is here that infectious agents such as bacteria and viruses first enter the fray. To describe this place appropriately, one must stoop to the cryptic and bilious language of darkness and melodrama. Enzymes are secreted by the pancreas and by cells in the crypts lining the long, serpentine halls. Bile from the liver enters the first part of the small intestine, the duodenum, and makes the fat soluble. Food that is broken down is ingested through the absorptive cells clustered on the folds, called villi, which, for bacteria, is the plural of *villa*, a great place to luxuriate.

Farther along, in the lower part of the ileum, most of the fluids and electrolytes mentioned earlier are absorbed. Few bacteria live naturally in the upper small intestine. Buffeted by peristaltic waves and rained upon with bile salts, they tend to move on in search of more hospitable environments. As well, the normal bacterial burghers of the lower small intestine fill up the available living space and effectively exclude, in most cases, all but the most aggressive newcomers. This phenomenon has been called competitive exclusion and is the rationale behind eating friendly bacteria, say, from yogurt, to prevent the pathogenic, disease-causing ones from moving into your neighborhood.

The small intestine is the central starting place for most foodborne illnesses. Nausea and vomiting, as in the stomach, still occur but are less common the farther into the bowels the intruders descend, at which point abdominal cramps and diarrhea predominate.

One group of bacteria, the *Yersinia* (related to the organism that causes human plague), has two members, *Y. enterocolitica* and *Y. pseudotuberculosis*, that are associated with food. In 1978, an intern from the Centers for Disease Control in Atlanta, Georgia, was going over records of appendectomies in Oneida County, New York. (This is the sort of sport in which an epidemiologist might engage during his or her spare time.) He found a definite peak in September 1976, and many of the sick kids came from a couple of small villages. His curiosity aroused, he dug deeper and found that in September and October of that year over two hundred children were sick with abdominal illness; thirty-six of them were hospitalized, and sixteen had appendectomies. This epidemic of apparent appendicitis was eventually traced back to chocolate milk provided in the school cafeteria. The milk was probably contaminated when the chocolate was mixed into the pasteurized milk in open vats. The ability to mimic appendicitis by infecting the tissues around the appendix is a particular trademark of this organism. People have succumbed to yersiniosis after drinking contaminated water or milk or eating a wide variety of foods, including tofu, chocolate syrup, raw pork, and—to put an old twist on an old saw—yellow snow.

While we are talking about what foodborne diseases do in the human gut, I must add something else: THERE IS NO SUCH DISEASE AS THE STOMACH FLU.

There. I have said it. When some viruses, with names like noroviruses and rotaviruses, invade the small intestine, they can cause diarrhea. Most of these viruses come from other peoples' butts. They get into water and into food, and they travel on handshakes. Not a nice thought. The flu vaccine won't protect you. Wash your hands.

Bacteria or viruses that manage to cause disease in the intestine often have special antigens, or proteins. Like specialized claws, these enable them to cling to the cell walls. Bacteria such as *Bacillus cereus, Clostridium perfringens,* and various strains of toxin-producing *E. coli* will attach themselves to the intestinal walls. There they multiply and produce toxins (called enterotoxins) that mimic the body's own secret code words (adenyl cyclase, for instance, will open a few doors), stimulating secretion of fluids into the intestines. Diarrhea and dehydration are the result.

Other bacteria or toxins such as *Salmonella,* if ingested in large numbers, may simply wreak wanton destruction on the cells lining the intestinal villi, even without attachment. In these cases, the food cannot be absorbed. Or the bacteria may themselves slip past the guards, invade the blood circulation, and knock the whole body back with a generalized illness (septicemia).

In some special cases, such as infant botulism, the normal, well-behaved bacterial citizens of the intestine have not yet moved in to set up shop, leaving their ecological niche wide open for opportunists. In other cases, antibiotics may be used, and like indiscriminate gut developers, they lay waste to particular ecological niches, where the pathogens can then multiply.

Parasites such as the tapeworms *Taenia saginata* and *Taenia solium* will attach themselves to the intestinal wall and feed, resulting in a chronic intestinal upset.

Many foodborne illnesses result from the absorption of toxins or viruses from the intestine into the blood; they do not cause disease in the gut itself but slip past the body's many defenses into the circuitous channels of blood to attack, say the liver (hepatitis A) or the nervous system (paralytic shellfish poisoning). Others, like the parasites *Toxoplasma* and *Trichinella,* enter the bloodstream and, like imperialistic Europeans, invade all parts of your body, starting small communities in the warm and nutritious New World of your flesh. The most serious foodborne toxins attack your nervous system, resulting in symptoms ranging from tingling, numbness, and vertigo to fatal paralysis.

In some cases, disease is caused not so much by the invader itself as by the immune response of the body. Hepatitis A doesn't usually cause serious disease in children, for instance, many of whom pick up the virus in day-care centers; children's immune systems are not well developed, and the viruses move in without causing major damage. The parents of kids from day-care centers are the ones at risk of getting very sick; when they get infected from their kids, their bodies attack the infected liver cells and they get jaundice.

With food allergies, the intruder may seem small and inoffensive, but the body engages in a vitriolic and self-destructive war against it. There are a variety of ways to get food allergies. If you expose enough people to a food intensively, over a long period, then some of them will get allergies. That is in part why peanut allergies occur in cultures where people eat lots of peanuts and milk allergies where people drink lots of milk. Foods that are described as "nonallergenic" in North America, and that are eaten by people with food allergies, may be common causes of allergies in other parts of the world.

Some food allergies may be acquired when your body is exposed to food molecules in unexpected ways. Let's say that you suffer a bout of bacterial diarrhea after eating undercooked shrimp. During your illness, your gut may be damaged, and some rather large shrimp molecules may barge their way across the wall from the lumen of the intestine (which, remember, is technically outside your body) into the inner sanctum of your blood and tissues. Your body, seeing these large, predigested shrimp molecules as foreigners, in the same general category as bacterial proteins, develops antibodies against them. The next time you eat shrimp, your body, thinking that a pre-emptive attack is called for, attacks the shrimp molecules even before they get down the gullet. Each time you are exposed, the reaction is stronger, as if your body has been stockpiling nuclear weapons in the interim. Before you know it, you are gasping for breath or dead.

In the early 1990s, I had a buffet meal with my family at a great local restaurant in St. Jacob's, Ontario. For dessert, I chose a piece of custard pie. Within minutes, I was kneeling before the butt-throne and throwing up. When I told the sweet girl behind the counter that the pie was bad, she was flustered and offered me another piece. "No," I told her. "It is *really* bad. It will give *lots* of people food poisoning. Probably *Staphylococcus aureus.*" She probably thought I was swearing and suggested that I wouldn't have to pay for the pie.

In the end, the restaurant gave me a free meal, but it was what came afterward that changed my life. The gut damage had allowed some larger molecules of egg to breach the intestinal walls and challenge my body's immune system to a lifelong fight. I have always loved making and eating foods with eggs in them: Spanish omelettes, huevos rancheros, chocolate cakes, soft-boiled eggs with a bit of butter and salt, waffles, crepes and pancakes, banana cream pie, chocolate cream pie, cheesecakes of all sorts, paska (traditional Mennonite Easter bread) with fresh orange frosting—the list is almost endless. At first, when I got queasy after eating eggs, I didn't think much of it. Then it was cakes.

One time my wife, Kathy, and I came home from the market with a piece of Greek layer cake. "This cake is bad," I said, running for the bathroom.

"It is?" said Kathy, reaching for a second piece.

Then I had scones at a restaurant that said they didn't have eggs in them. I cured that by emptying my stomach into the plumbing system and making myself some chicken noodle soup. That was when I discovered that the noodles in chicken noodle soup have eggs in them. The last two times I reacted was when someone at Tim Horton's assured me that their bread had no eggs in it and I just about died in the parking lot as my lungs filled with water, and on a trail in Bruce County, after having some homemade chocolate from a local store. From the Tim Horton's episode, I learned that baking prepared in a donut-making factory probably has some egg in it. From the chocolate episode, I discovered that lecithin, an emulsifier used in some chocolates, may be from vegetable (usually soy) or other (sometimes egg) sources.

I now carry an EpiPen (injectable adrenaline) and have to go through long explanations in airports to people who understand as much about foodborne diseases and allergies as the girl behind the restaurant counter did. I also carry antihistamines, which, if I use them as soon as I suspect there might be a problem, can head off the worst effects. Once, in Addis Ababa, I was worried about the ingredients of the food I had eaten, so I took some of the bright pink Benadryl pills I had in my pocket. I had a rough-and-tumble stomach all night. The next morning, I discovered that the pink pills I had swallowed were not antihistamines but a cathartic (an antidote to constipation). I guessed that there had been no eggs in what I had eaten, or I would not have survived the night.

I could likely sue the restaurant owner, but he's an acquaintance, so I haven't even told him. Which is probably irresponsible of me. Instead, I have my students prepare public dissemination projects and hammer into them the public part of public health. And I write books like this one.

At least one kind of food intoxication mimics an allergic reaction. Sometimes, in scombroid fish such as tuna and in some cheeses, bacteria may partly digest the food (some might call it spoilage, but I am trying not to be judgmental). When eaten in large amounts, such spoiled foods cause symptoms that may be confused with those of true allergies: a burning in the mouth and throat, flushing, and dizziness.

In early March of 1981, a young, organized British Columbia woman bought two cases of canned tuna. She opened a can
from the first case and ate the contents, despite their strange,
bitter taste, on March 15. About half an hour later, she felt
nauseated, her throat was swelling, and she felt hot; she also
developed what appeared to be a rash on her chest and back.
On March 22, probably thinking about fiscal responsibility and
the large investment she had just made in tuna, she tried again,
with the same results. Almost exactly nine years later, three
people in downtown Toronto tried out a local luncheon special
of mahimahi fish. Within the next hour, all three felt as if they
had a sudden sunburn. Peppery taste, headache, dizziness, diarrhea, and flushing are recognized symptoms of food allergies.

At one time, scombroid fish poisoning was thought to be a
kind of allergy. Now we know that it is neither an allergy nor
restricted to scombroid fish such as tuna, mackerel, and other
dark-fleshed fish, like mahimahi. Scombroid "fish" poisoning
has also been reported from eating Swiss cheese. Some bacteria
will digest foods containing the amino acid histidine, such as
fish that have not been cleaned and chilled quickly enough. The
product of the bacteria's labor is histamine, the same compound
made by our own bodies during an allergic reaction—hence the
similarities in clinical picture. The big difference, however, is
that our bodies learn from a food allergy. One encounter, however benign, enhances the seriousness of the next. Scombroid
toxicity is more like a predictable aunt, with unchanged irritability from visit to visit.

In both neurological and allergic-type reactions, ordinary
citizens might ascribe their state to a stimulating dinner companion, were it not followed so inconveniently by more serious
gastrointestinal or neurological complications.

Foodborne illnesses may also result from food intolerances,
in which case your body does not have the enzymes necessary

to digest certain parts of certain foods. Milk intolerance is a common problem among some ethnic groups, which results in frothy diarrhea and cramps. Many of us can recall stories of poor villagers in some developing country using powdered milk to whitewash their houses. One might view this use as a form of ingratitude in the face of our obvious generosity, but such generosity is not much different from their sending us skewered cockroaches to solve our food problems. Another food intolerance, this one found in many people of Mediterranean origin, is called favism. These people can develop an acute hemolytic anemia if they eat fava beans.

The large intestine is mostly a place where fluids and electrolytes get sucked back into your body. Being less acidic than other parts of your gut, the large intestine is generally hospitable to bacteria, many of which normally make their home there and don't cause illness. In fact, one might suggest that the only ecological and evolutionary justification for the human race is to serve as a living area for large numbers of anaerobic (air-intolerant) bacteria. This perception is not as heady as thinking of ourselves as the brains of evolution, but in ecologically recessionary times, when millions of species are going extinct for lack of a working niche, it is at least a job. The total number of bacteria excreted by an adult each day ranges from a hundred billion to a hundred trillion.

If pathogenic agents do manage to get a foothold in these nether regions, we feel lower abdominal cramps and can develop bloody diarrhea. Red blood in the feces is a sign that the destruction must be quite low down, because blood entering the intestines higher up turns black through partial digestion.

Finally, high-fiber foods such as bran will draw water into the large intestine and smuggle it away to the great outdoors in what is called an osmotic diarrhea.

The foregoing are the acute effects of foodborne diseases. These diseases may also have long-term effects, sometimes called sequelae. Reactive arthritis develops in more than 6 percent of people who get salmonellosis and in probably 1 percent of those with *Campylobacter* infection. *Campylobacter* infections can be followed by Guillain-Barré syndrome, in which people develop burning sensations and paralysis; 15 percent of them die. There is also some evidence that foodborne infections may contribute to plaques in blood vessels and hence to cardiovascular disease. Diseases caused by *E. coli* O157:H7 (so-called hamburger disease) can lead to chronic kidney failure or chronic bowel diseases. Some kinds of fish and shellfish poisonings result in chronic neurological and memory problems (that's my excuse for forgetting things).

So, you have survived the journey; to paraphrase an ancient Persian saying, the fine wine of France has been transformed by the human body into urine, and the succulent cabbage rolls of Kiev have been transformed into fertilizer. Millions of bacteria have died. Millions more have been born. Whole civilizations have come and gone in the bowels of your body. Truly, a Wagnerian chorus could not match the richness of this drama.

WHEN SHE STAYS

FOR

BREAKFAST

3

SALMONELLA

READING

IN

TURKEY

FOODBORNE INFECTIONS,

FOCUSING ON SALMONELLA

T O SOMEONE not well versed in the literature on food poisoning, the title of this chapter might sound like a headline in a supermarket tabloid about a literate fish discovered in Istanbul. In fact, the report that carried this title described an outbreak of gastrointestinal disease among hospital food-service employees related to infection with a particular strain of the bacteria *Salmonella* first recognized in Reading, England, and therefore named after that place. *Salmonella* are often named after the places where they were first discovered. If the *Salmonella* were to have their own family picnic, there would be some 2,500 of them, from all over the world. There are *Salmonella* named after Aberdeen and Adelaide, Caracas and Dublin, all the way down

41

the alphabet to Zanzibar. These names could result in mind-bending medical headlines, involving, say, *Salmonella uganda* invading New York. Microbiologists have recently tried to remedy this problem by giving all the *Salmonella* that attack the gut a middle name, *enterica*. This system may please the classifiers, but it doesn't do much for those who just want to give their gut problems a proper name. In this book, I have stuck with the old names, just because they require fewer words.

If we take a global view of our existence on this planet—that is, that we are all part of the living, breathing organism that British scientist James Lovelock has called Gaia—then the bacteria, parasites, and even natural toxins that make us sick are as much at home here as we are. They are not here to make us sick, any more than we are here to destroy the rain forests. If evolutionary microbiologist Lynn Margulis is correct, then people are entirely composed of various kinds of bacteria, and each of us is a synergistic colony of microbes, a cross between priest-archeologist Teilhard de Chardin's grandiose vision of the universe becoming God and an amazing, lumbering grade-B horror movie attempt of the universe to understand itself. "What a piece of work is man!" said Shakespeare. Indeed.

The sicknesses we suffer are a side effect of an imbalance in human-microbial relations, some distortion in our collective ecosystem, resulting in the migration of disease-causing microbes from their natural homes into our food, and from there into our bodies. More often than not, the ecosystem distortion or cause of the bacterial migration is human in origin. Perhaps the easiest way to explore foodborne infections as a complex social-ecological issue is to look closely at the emergence and behavior of *Salmonella* epidemics over the past few decades.

On June 24, 1984, a seventy-one-year-old lady went to a family picnic in Moncton, New Brunswick. Little did she know, when she ate her morsel of cheese, that she was to be part of a great Canadian historical event, celebrated in bacterial circles and rued in milk producers' circles for many years to come. On June 27, this modest, grandmotherly woman came down with nausea and diarrhea. Although some folks have been known to react in similar fashion to family picnics, this woman did not think family events were quite that bad. On June 28, she started vomiting; by June 30, things were getting worse, and she ended up in the hospital, from which she emerged shaken but alive on July 5.

That same day, the cheese manufacturer, in Prince Edward Island, issued a national recall of its products, which were distributed across Canada under various brand names. What the woman in Moncton did not know was that she was near the tail end of a six-month epidemic of salmonellosis that attacked more than two thousand people in the Maritimes and Ontario. The investigation of this epidemic, the largest of its kind in Canada, had progressed more slowly than it should have for various reasons. Not all the investigators saw the value of sound epidemiologic methods and did not always include a comparison, or control group, in their investigations. Cheese was not always considered a real food by those who got sick; they thought of it as a snack and thus did not include it in their food history questionnaire. The cheese involved was distributed to most Canadian provinces under eighteen brand names, making it difficult to trace. Finally, the number of bacteria in the cheese was very low. One Canadian researcher estimated, based on a series of case studies, that people in this epidemic got sick by eating fewer than half a dozen of these microscopic bacteria.

The organism involved in this epidemic, a strain of *Salmonella typhimurium,* was traced back to the factory where the cheese was made. There, it turned out, one of the workers decided to turn off some valves manually, even though an electronically controlled flow-diversion valve was in place. As a result, raw milk that was supposed to go to the pasteurizer ended up in the cheese vat, and 2,700 people got sick. The milk with the *Salmonella* in it was traced to one teat on one cow on one farm. She was a good producer, but she had chronic mastitis, not caused by *Salmonella,* although she was shedding it.

Most of the agents that cause food poisoning have a natural home—that is, they have evolved a niche for themselves where, like most of us, they carry out their recycling and respiratory functions with minimal trauma to their immediate neighbors. Over the years, a high proportion of outbreaks of foodborne disease in Canada and the United States has been traced to chicken, turkey, pork, and beef. Other *Salmonella* prefer pigeons, gulls, and people.

As in any respectable family, there are a few black sheep and troublemakers that will stir up a good gut incident no matter where they are. However, in its natural home setting, *Salmonella* organisms, like most of the agents that cause foodborne disease, often live like good quiet farmers in the hinterlands of their chosen animal hosts. The Maritime cow with the bacteria dripping from her teat is typical.

That year, 1984, George Orwell's year of doom, was a bad year for salmonellosis in Canada. In September 1984, for instance, the Pope helicoptered in to visit the Jesuit mission of Sainte-Marie among the Hurons near Midland, Ontario. Of the more than sixteen hundred police officers who provided security, five hundred ate the roast beef boxed lunch offered by volunteers. Within the next twenty-four hours, as they headed home, just about every one of those police officers got sick. Newspaper reports describe police sick with severe diarrhea and vomiting on buses and motorcycles, finding bathrooms where they could, running from squad cars into the woods. In the weeks that followed, twenty-seven (over 6 percent) of the infected officers developed reactive (secondary) arthritis—pain and swelling in many of their joints. Some of them ended up with permanent joint damage. This painful arthritis, which is sometimes associated with eye and urinary tract inflammation, is a known consequence of infections with foodborne organisms such as *Salmonella, Campylobacter,* and *Yersinia.* Reactive arthritis used to be called Reiter's syndrome, after the physician who discovered it in 1916. Unfortunately, Dr. Reiter later went on to a less-than-glorious career doing experiments in the Nazi death camps—hence the new name for the disease.

The 1984 outbreaks in Canada were a sign of things to come from the *Salmonella* gang. In the spring of 1985, some 16,000 people in and around Chicago were reported to have acquired *Salmonella*-associated diarrhea and vomiting after a small technical mix-up in a dairy processing plant. After an intensive investigation, the estimate of casualties was raised to almost 200,000. Only a few months before, the plant had been hailed as one of the safest and most modern in the United States (and by implication, of course, the world). In this case the cause appeared to be a structural flaw in the technology itself, which, as in Prince Edward Island, had allowed some unpasteurized milk to slip into the system. After the epidemic the plant, the largest in U.S. history until then, went bankrupt.

In 1994 an estimated 224,000 people got sick from *Salmonella typhimurium.* Tanker trucks in Minnesota that had been carrying liquid raw eggs were subsequently used to haul ice cream premix. The tanks had apparently not been well cleaned out. All the eggs were in one basket and guess what? Somebody dropped it.

When I'm teaching, I like to tell the parallel story, which also took place in 1994, of the old Mennonite couple at the St. Jacobs farmers' market who sold a homemade delicacy called cook cheese. Apparently, they didn't properly clean out a barrel that had been used to store chickens. Eighty-two people got sick. It was big news locally. It was sad for the old couple, but the problem could be handled locally and provided an excellent opportunity for education. There are still many such small outbreaks around the world. The major advantage, from a public health point of view, is that you can identify the farms, talk to the farmers, and improve the situation with a few simple recommendations. Trace-backs, responses, and regulations are much more difficult at economies of scale; they require more sophisticated (and expensive) molecular laboratory techniques and tend to evoke industrial-type solutions, like food irradiation, which mostly increase problems rather than solve them.

Several other trends have emerged in recent years. First, even if they are not large, outbreaks of salmonellosis and other foodborne bacteria are becoming more widespread as they cross borders and oceans. We are in the midst of a Salmonella pandemic. Because of mass distribution of food, and because food from many sources gets mixed up, relabeled, and redistributed at various points in the system, outbreaks are more difficult to trace back to where they started. Second, even though the bacteria involved are considered to be adapted to animals, they are also being connected with fresh produce. The sh*t is everywhere: fresh sprouts of all sorts, cantaloupe, chip dips, minced beef, powdered milk, lettuce, tomatoes, and pigs' ears (fed as treats to dogs that then infect people) are some of the sources of human infections. Finally, some of the newer strains of *Salmonella* are resistant to a wide variety of antibiotics.

Salmonella typhimurium DT104, which sounds like the name of a small warship, first emerged in cattle in the United Kingdom in the early 1980s and then went pandemic in the next couple of decades. This organism is more likely to kill both people and animals than other members of the *Salmonella* extended family and is resistant to most of the antibacterial drugs one might wish to launch against it. Fortunately, although it has become widespread in North America and Europe, it does not (yet) appear to be common.

Trying to understand the emergence and spread of *Salmonella* is a lesson in the complex dynamics of social-ecological systems we think we control. Although a few of them prefer one host (*typhi* in people, *cholerae-suis* in pigs), most *Salmonella* are both liberated and cosmopolitan. S. *panama* came into the United Kingdom by way of dried eggs during World War II and from there migrated into pig feed and from there into people. S. *eastbourne* rode the cocoa bean boats from Africa into eastern Canada and brought its sweet tenesmus dances to children all over Canada and the United States in contaminated candy. Among the many we might reflect upon, the story of *Salmonella enteritidis* may be one of the more instructive.

Chickens and turkeys often carry a few *Salmonella* in their intestines or on their feathers, without any apparent ill effects. Tens of millions of people have gotten sick from similarly few *Salmonella* over the past few decades, and many have died. We are currently on the slowly declining tail (we hope) of a global pandemic of salmonellosis, mostly from chickens and mostly S. *enteritidis*. But bacteria are, from an evolutionary point of view, considerably more "fit" than the rest of us, and the emergence of S. *enteritidis* furnishes a cautionary tale.

In the early twentieth century, two serologically related *Salmonellas*—S. *gallinarum*, which causes diarrhea in chicks, and S. *pullorum*, or fowl typhoid, were quite common in poultry flocks in Europe and North America. Veterinarians noticed two important things about these organisms: they were adapted to domestic chickens and waterfowl, and they made the birds (but not people) sick. The first characteristic made the disease vulnerable to a "test and slaughter" method of eradication—a kind of mass-slaughter/napalm operation that many animal disease control people seem to find attractive (someone should do a psychological study on that); the second characteristic was strong motivation to carry out such a program. The eradication of fowl typhoid has been a success story; the disease is rare in any country that boasts a "modern" poultry industry.

About the same time as this *Salmonella* was eliminated from poultry, another *Salmonella*—S. *enteritidis*—wandered over from its natural home in rodents and took up residence in the vacated ecological niche. Not many disease specialists know much about ecology, so this shift in bacterial ecology was not widely investigated. The notion that various species of all types and sizes in the world are interconnected, and that ecological niches are not really vacated but just filled with other species, makes disease treatment and control seem, well, complicated.

In any case, the vets didn't worry too much about it, since *enteritidis* doesn't make chickens sick. It does make people sick, however, but veterinarians and physicians have a long history of not talking much to each other. By the late 1980s, there was a global pandemic—in people, not chickens. *Enteritidis* was even more clever than scientists imagined, since it lived inside the ovaries of the birds laying the eggs, and they got it from their closely guarded and very valuable parents, the so-called breeder flocks. These flocks are the source of most of the world's commercial chickens. People didn't even have to be dirty to get sick. All that hand washing and all those chemicals for naught! All those great genetics! How could a bacterium be so vile and anarchistic?

In 1988, Edwina Currie, then a junior health minister in the British government, drew attention to a problem with S. *enteritidis* in eggs. After Edwina made her announcement, sales of eggs in the UK fell by 60 percent overnight, and many egg producers went out of business; Edwina herself was relieved of her job. By 1994, Edwina was back in the news, helping to launch a celebrity-chef cookbook called *My Perfect Omelette* and claiming that British eggs were now the safest in the world. That may well be, but the global pandemic of salmonellosis is not over yet, and the organisms keep coming up with new chemical-evading stratagems as fast as those chemicals can be devised.

S. *enteritidis* continues to adapt. An epidemic in Canada and the United States of an unusual molecular strain, PT 30, was traced to raw whole almonds in 2000 and 2001. (The PT refers to "phage type"; phages are viruses that infect bacteria and can be used to trace them.) PT 30 is an uncommon strain in foodborne diseases, and almonds are an uncommon vehicle for infection. Investigators looked everywhere for an animal source, since *Salmonella* are not supposed to live out there in the wild without an animal host. They couldn't find any animals near the nut farms. One of the researchers has suggested that the bacteria have been growing in the soil, which, because the almond growers have been growing trees at much higher densities than was once thought possible, is richer in nutrients than was once thought possible. If this supposition is true, then people have pushed the bacteria down new, interesting, and (for consumers) dangerous evolutionary paths.

Most *Salmonella* do not travel first class, as the ones inside the eggs have. Usually, they hang around in the dust and feces in the chicken barn, cling to the outside of the eggshell, and only get into the eggs after the eggshells have been washed. A 2006 survey in Europe found that in some countries, such as the Czech Republic, Poland, and Spain, more than 70 percent of egg-laying flocks are infected with *Salmonella*. With the exception of the Nordic countries (which have all but eradicated the disease in animals), other industrialized countries have lower, but still substantial, levels of contamination. In washing the eggs, people remove not only the visible dirt but also the less visible protective layer that the hen has secreted over her baby's shell. The invisible bacteria are left intact and ready to invade through the pores of the egg, which they do as the shell dries.

Salmonella in cattle may move from the rural backwoods of intestinal living to adopt suburban lifestyles in lymph nodes. Even people can carry the organisms without being sick. Mary Malone, the infamous cook called Typhoid Mary, was one of many such people who have spread infections without themselves being sick. How we deal with such people (or animals) raises all the great questions of private rights versus public good that are at the heart of public health. Should people be quarantined? Cautioned? Charged with mischief?

A few bacteria do not usually cause much of a problem. What brings the masses out into the streets, however, is stress. Crowding the chickens or pigs together, and piling them into trucks to go to the slaughterhouse, brings *Salmonella* into the bracing, rebellious air, infiltrating feathers, splotching skin, and multiplying and filling the earth. If animals are not contaminated before they get into the truck to go to slaughter, they probably are afterward. Various studies find significant degrees of contamination in retail meats in Canada, the United States, and Europe (with the exception of the Nordic countries). Even if the prevalence gets down to, say, 1 percent, you, as a consumer, don't know which 1 percent that is.

With all the scalds and disinfectants in modern packing plants, a lot of bacteria on the chickens do meet their end at the slaughterhouse. But with the crowds out full force, there are always a few million to spare, and bacteria love to multiply. Some of those millions get siphoned off into the meat by-products and from there get into the animal feeds and go back to the quiet life on the farm. The rest of them head off to the bright city lights, weddings, family reunions, papal visits, hospitals, and nursing homes.

From the point of view of the bacteria, bigger is better; the more intensive and large scale the livestock operations, the more extensive and devastating the foodborne disease, as well as the ecological problems. *Salmonella* in the family cow no longer need to content themselves with recycling through the same boring small family but get a free ride across the country and around the world. The notion of bacteria coming through in the eggs really only becomes frightening when one considers that a few major companies supply all the source birds for the egg industry. Monocultures and world trade are tailor-made for bacterial survival: the economies of scale are the economics of pandemics.

Another way to help the *Salmonella* along at the farm is to feed the animals antibiotics, which kill off the other neighborhood bacteria. The hardy and often drug-resistant *Salmonella*, never being ones to waste an opportunity, move into the homes we have cleaned out with our preemptive public safety measures. This tactic also works at home; you can sometimes lure a latent case of salmonellosis out of the closet by taking penicillin. Because of the massive amounts of antibiotics used in both people and animals, some people fear that drug-resistant *Salmonella* might take over the world. Drug-resistant bacteria, however, are adapted to live in a drug-filled environment, and if we cut back on our profligate antibiotic use, they would not give us problems.

If the bacteria can almost count on a quiet home on the farm, opportunities to spread from animal to animal abound on the truck to market. Even more opportunities arise at slaughter, and they most certainly can look forward to sloppiness in the kitchen. The counter becomes contaminated with bacteria when the turkey is put down there for dressing. Those that accompany the bird into the oven usually get killed off, but a healthy population lurks on the counter and repopulates it. If the counter is not contaminated, then your hands, or the knives, are. (What do you do about that itch on your scalp just before you handle the dinner? Just a little scratch won't hurt, will it?) It is best, from a bacterial point of view, if you let the meat sit on the counter for a while, just to incubate.

Salmonella get turned on by that sort of warm, moist situation. They tumble over themselves in incestuous delight, doubling their populations every half hour or so. Other bacteria are even speedier. *E. coli*, a common gut bacterium, doubles every fifteen to twenty minutes, and *Clostridium perfringens*, which tends to favor meaty gravies and causes a passing diarrhea, is a copulatory sprinter at an eight- to ten-minute doubling time. I am told by a microbiologist colleague that, with unlimited food and ideal warmth, one cell could multiply to a colony of clones four thousand times the mass of the earth in twenty-four hours. Fortunately, the cells run out of food before they reach that size.

If poultry are a haven for *Salmonella*, hamburgers are heaven for a veritable menagerie of bacteria. Bacteria generally sit on the surface of meat, which includes the turkey's armpits but not the heart of a steak. When we make hamburger, we take the surface bacteria and integrate them into the larger community of meat. Hamburgers, then, are really just cases of diarrhea and vomiting waiting for stomachs to happen, unless you cook them, and cook them well. Some of America's finest foodborne disease outbreaks have been tracked back to hamburgers.

Like most of us, *Salmonella* prefer temperatures that are warm but not hot and will survive freezing but not boiling. They abhor the caustic wit of bleach and the acidic tongue of tomato juice, but they are adaptable enough to make a go of it in the most soiled of environments.

Hopelessness in the face of universal pollution is sometimes used as an argument by polluters to continue polluting; in the case of antibiotic resistance in bacteria, however, the situation is not at all hopeless. Bacteria can change rapidly; the same characteristics that allow them to develop antimicrobial resistance will also lead them to drop much of that resistance. Not burdened with rules of socially acceptable reproductive behavior, they can evolve and adapt as quickly to a drug-free life as they have to drugs. If Solomon had advised us to go to the bacteria, where quick, guiltless, cooperative change is the watchword, instead of to the ants, where regimented war prevails, who knows what the shape of human civilization might be today? The short of it is: things will get better if we change our ways.

Countries such as Sweden and Denmark have been systematic and aggressive in addressing *Salmonella* problems. Through a mixture of legal requirements and commercial inducements, *Salmonella* has been reduced and all but eradicated on farms, at slaughterhouses, and in the human population in these countries. So improvements are possible, but they are going to take some realistic, complex, systems thinking, firm commitments, and perhaps some deep cultural changes. For some of us, becoming more Swedish would, after all, not be so bad.

4

COWS, CATS,

AND

PURE COUNTRY

WATER

E. COLI AND OTHER WATERBORNE

BACTERIAL INFECTIONS

DRINKING BOTTLED water every day is like using a toilet bowl brush to clean your teeth, driving a snowmobile for recreation, or using an all-terrain vehicle in the city. All these items have important uses, but in most parts of the world none of them should be part of everyday life. When they are used outside of the circumstance for which they are designed, they are, for the most part, destructive and dysfunctional. Bottled water is for emergencies and should be saved for them.

Mostly, I dislike bottled water because it represents an unwarranted and pervasive anxiety in Western societies. Bottled water purports to solve an individual problem—fear of illness—by contributing unnecessarily to big public health problems—large-scale water and energy shortages and under-funded public water systems. I hate the idea that someone can suck an increasingly scarce public good out of the ground and then use scarce energy resources to package it and sell it back to the public. This process fosters an obsession with personal health, even as it puts the health of our children in jeopardy by undermining the health of the ecosystems that provide the basis for all life. The money spent on bottled water would be better spent on improving public water systems.

Bottled water may or may not be safer than tap water. The jury is out on that. Because any disease outbreaks caused by bottled water would be widely dispersed and not likely linked by individuals or physicians to that plastic-wrapped water on the counter, they would not very likely be identified. Because most people see bottled water as a solution rather than a problem, there's not much in the literature. In 1993, two babies were brought into a Wisconsin hospital having seizures; the seizures were caused by intoxication with low-sodium bottled water, the mother having apparently thought that bottled water was better for her babies than tap water. In 2000, the Centers for Disease Control and Prevention reported that it had detected a ten-state bottled-water-associated outbreak of salmonellosis through a special pattern-recognition program called the *Salmonella* Outbreak Detection Algorithm, or SODA for short. A report in the journal *Emerging Infectious Diseases* identified bottled water as one of the risk factors for *Campylobacter* infection in the United Kingdom.

I am not a fanatic about bottled water. It obviously makes sense in natural disasters, such as the sudden floods in Vancouver (probably related to global warming) in the fall of 2006. I used to carry water bottles onto airplanes, where the air is very dry, but since August 2006, this has become impossible. I don't mind, as long as water is readily available on the plane. I occasionally carry bottled water in the car or on hikes. If I have bought a bottle of water, I always refill it from the tap, a practice that bottled water companies warn me against, as they suggest it might lead to contamination.

I often drink bottled carbonated water in parts of Africa, Asia, and Latin America, where public funding for clean water has been scarce (usually as the result of development or financial or trade programs instigated by financial institutions based in North America or Europe). I drink the carbonated stuff because the nonbubbly bottled water, in whatever country you live, is often no better than the water out of the tap. In most countries, however, including nominally Muslim countries, I prefer the beer (which I know uses a lot of water).

The bottled water industry thrives on a public fear of contaminated water, and I really don't like any industry that thrives on fear, especially fear that I have contributed to, which, by teaching about food- and waterborne diseases, I probably have. If this chapter on waterborne disease drives you to drink bottled water rather than to advocate for better public water systems, then I have failed.

So let me start by confronting the fear.

In May 2000, the small rural town of Walkerton, Ontario (population about 5,000), hit the international headlines. I remember the day, because a friend called me into the common room at the Makerere University Guest House in Kampala, Uganda, to tell me that Canada was in the news. People were dying from drinking tap water.

It started with a few reports of cases of bloody diarrhea in nursing homes and schools and ended with more than 2,300 people sick. Twenty-seven people had to be hospitalized with hemolytic uremic syndrome, a rare disease involving the breakdown of red blood cells, blood in the urine, and kidney failure. At least six people died. Some of my best friends and colleagues (veterinarians and graduates of our epidemiology program at Guelph) led the public health investigations, so I got a variety of inside and outside stories. The outbreak led to one of the most thorough inquiries into a public health disaster in Canadian history.

The drinking water for a large part of the town had been contaminated with two organisms: vero-toxin producing *E. coli*, or VTEC (pronounced vee-tek) for short, and *Campylobacter*. The most common type of VTEC is also called O157:H7, the O referring to some proteins on the surface of its body, and the H to proteins on its tail. Other *E. coli*'s produce the same kind of toxin, but O157:H7 is the most famous. The toxin, also called shigatoxin because it is the same one produced by *Shigella*, which causes bloody dysentery in travelers and people who live in poor neighborhoods, kills kidney cells from African green monkeys (vero cells). There must be a good reason that the laboratory people picked exactly those cells to test toxins in—some dislike of African green monkeys perhaps. The green monkeys wrought their revenge by inflicting a hemorrhagic illness called Marburg disease on some of the lab workers, but that is another story.

In one sense, the presence of these organisms in water systems in rural areas was not surprising. Our research group at Guelph had identified rural areas and areas with denser cattle populations that spread manure on farmland as having higher rates of *E. coli*-related infections than urban areas. We'd already had one tragic outbreak in Ontario related to a well-run farm, in 1986. It was a typical Ontario farm, with sixty-seven cows and calves, some chickens, and some pigs, all well cared for and clean, and seemed the perfect place to take your class of preschoolers. In April of that year, sixty-two preschool children and twelve supervising adults visited this farm. They played in the barn, petted the calves, pulled at the cows' teats, and gathered a few eggs. For a break, they drank milk (right from the farmer's tank!) and ate egg cookies (sliced hard-boiled eggs cleverly renamed to induce children to eat them). A good time was had by all.

Within the next two weeks, forty-two children and four adults came down with abdominal cramps and diarrhea. Three of the children ended up in hospital with hemolytic uremic syndrome. One of the children fell into a coma. All eventually recovered.

The public health investigators looked everywhere on the farm. Although they found only two calves carrying the organism, they decided that exposure to the unpasteurized milk was the most plausible explanation for what they saw. And yet the farm family, which drank that milk every day, was apparently healthy and not shedding VTEC. Since that time, VTEC had been found to live comfortably and usually without any harmful side effects in the intestines of many cattle, just about wherever cattle are raised, at least in industralized countries.

Campylobacter, particularly *C. jejuni,* the other organism found in the water at Walkerton, has been found in many of the same waterborne outbreaks as *E. coli. Campylobacter* is the bug of choice for cooks, college students, drinkers of raw milk, and, if the aforementioned study in the United Kingdom is to be believed, bottled-water drinkers.

Although reports of so-called intestinal flu involving curvaceous wiggling organisms in milk go back to 1946, the first major review of *Campylobacter jejuni* as a possible common cause of diarrhea in people only appeared in the scientific literature in 1977. Just about everywhere researchers have looked for it, they have found it; it is at home in most warm-blooded animals but seems to have a fondness for birds. Today most researchers consider it the most common cause of bacterial diarrhea in the United Kingdom and in North America.

Campylobacter does not grow very well in food, which is why it causes disease in those who handle raw food, such as cooks. College students, especially those who eat chicken and live with cats, were shown in one study to be a high-risk group. This is related to the "second weaning" phenomenon; those poor suckers are just learning how to cook and they discover that what looked easy when Mom and Dad did it actually requires some skill. Symptoms of the disease—diarrhea, abdominal pain, headache, fever, bloody stools, nausea, and sometimes vomiting—start up to a week after the offending meal and last a week. The reason some of these infections take so long to develop is that the bacteria make their way down to the large intestine before setting up shop, multiplying like mad, and making trouble. That's also why you see actual blood in the stools of infected people; if the infection is higher up, in the small intestine, the blood is digested and you see black tarry stuff coming out.

Like *Salmonella, Campylobacter* doesn't just cause immediate damage to the gut. Some victims get reactive arthritis I described in the section about salmonellosis. About one in a thousand of those infected with *Campylobacter* go on to develop a paralytic disease called Guillain-Barré syndrome.

Campylobacter grows best at about 108°F, which is quite warm. That is why it is often associated with birds, which have a higher internal temperature than us mammals. In one study in the United Kingdom, milk bottles that had been attacked by free-enterprising starlings at the doorstep were found to be a source of infection for people. The birds followed the milk delivery truck and then poked through the tops of the bottles for a fresh drink. Although *Campylobacter* grows best in birds, it has been isolated from river and sea water, mud, sewage, and sludge.

This disease appears to be most serious in Western peoples living under conditions of good hygiene. In many developing countries, it seems to be found almost as often in healthy people as in sick people. Clinically normal animals in all countries can carry the organism. In people in developing countries, and in farm animals in North America, the organism can be found with just about equal frequency in healthy and diarrheic individuals.

Although infection is common, disease, in adults at least, does not appear to be as common as would be expected, suggesting that immunity might be developed by continuous exposure.

One study has shown that college students who visited a friend's home farm got sick from drinking the milk, while the farm family remained cheerfully healthy. One of the costs, then, of protecting children from disease is that, as adults, they are more vulnerable. The alternative, however—to expose kids while young and let the strongest survive—is hardly tenable morally.

Overall, the presence of VTEC in cows and *Campylobacter* in a variety of animals didn't explain the Walkerton outbreak. I visited the farm from which, allegedly, the offending organisms entered the city's water system. It was run by a veterinarian just outside the town limits. It was no factory farm. Like the farm in the center of the 1986 tragedy, it was an idyllic place, with some corn and a few cows, the kind of place held up as a perfect example of all those who want a return to the simple life of small family farms. The farmer had in place a good Environmental Farm Plan, a program devised by Ontario farmers to assess how well they are managing the landscapes of which they are stewards.

There are a lot of bad things a person could say about feedlots and factory farms, and I would be one of the first to voice them, but the Walkerton outbreak cannot be laid at that door. The outbreak represented a failure to think systemically; it was a triumph of boundaries, blinders, governmental departmental silos, and small-mindedness. The farm was just outside city limits, so the ecologically important boundaries did not match the political decision-making boundaries. The contaminated well was located on low ground, apparently in a place that engineers had advised against but that made short-term economic sense. The provincial government was ideologically driven and reckless, typical of both communist and free enterprise governments the world over. It cut back on environmental programs, privatized laboratory testing, and downloaded responsibilities without paying attention to whether local officials were up to those responsibilities. The guy who was supposed to monitor water quality didn't know anything about water quality, drank on the job, and fabricated data. Nobody seemed to be quite sure who was supposed to report to whom or who was ultimately responsible. Because of all the government cutbacks, no one was watching. The government seemed more concerned about building highways, encouraging the trucking industry, and dismissing the values of higher education than they were about public health.

In the week before the tragedy, rainfall in the Walkerton area exceeded the amount expected no more than once every half a century to a century. Such extreme rainfalls are known to occur under conditions of global warming, which is encouraged by more highways, more trucking, and cavalier economists and politicians who know very little about biology and could not care less about public health. Heavy rainfall preceded an outbreak of waterborne disease in Milwaukee, Wisconsin, in 1993. That one, involving the single-celled animal parasite, Cryptosporidium, affected more than 400,000 people and killed more than 50 of them. Since the Walkerton episode, several studies in both Canada and the United States, including some by members of our group in Guelph, have confirmed this relationship between heavy rainfall and disease outbreaks. Does this surprise us? You put manure out on the land, the rainfall flushes it, you drink, you get sick. In many parts of the world, global warming means more extreme droughts followed by heavier rainfalls, which is comparable to not flushing for a while and then, well, you get the picture.

I have introduced *E. coli* as a waterborne disease, because in many cases that is what it has become. With agricultural intensification and encroachment of urban settlements into rural areas, the organism is now, like *Salmonella*, widespread in the food system. Between 1995 and 2006, eighteen outbreaks of *E. coli* O157:H7 in the United States were linked to lettuce. In 2006, almost two hundred people were made sick in Canada and the United States by contaminated spinach. Much of the contaminated produce was traced back to a valley in California. It is worthwhile to remember that it wasn't always this way and to consider a little of the recent history of how VTEC made its way into public consciousness.

The first report of an outbreak of human disease caused by VTEC, in 1982, was titled "Hemorrhagic colitis associated with a rare *Escherichia coli* serotype." Forty-seven people came down with the disease—"grossly bloody diarrhea," the report called it (is there a fine bloody diarrhea?). All had eaten beef patties at a restaurant chain in Michigan and Oregon. That same year, there was a report from a children's hospital in Toronto that hemolytic uremic syndrome, a kidney disease that results in bloody urine, was connected to drinking fresh apple juice. Before then, no one had made the connection. A few years later, there were outbreaks in nursing homes, summer camps, schools, and petting zoos. By 1988, Dr. Lester Crawford, Administrator of the Food Safety and Inspection Service in the United States, in what sounded like a cry of panic, called it "the most dangerous food poisoning organism known to man."

The best way to have an outbreak in a food is to declare that food safe. The North American public has been told repeatedly by food industry experts that it has the safest food system in the world. At the same time, so-called hamburger disease has been transmitted by unpasteurized milk; ham, turkey, or cheese sandwiches; raw apple juice; natural apple cider; wheat noodles; fresh produce, and water. In 1991, 520 people in the Northwest Territories got sick from O157:H7 and 2 people died. The median age of the sick people was six years. The original food source wasn't identified, and there seemed to be a lot of person-to-person spread once the epidemic got started. This epidemic never made the headlines, and not much came of it; someone less kind than me might suggest that this was because the victims were Inuit.

Just over a year later, in late 1992 and early 1993, about the same number of children got sick. But this time the victims were kids in Washington State who had eaten hamburgers at a well-known fast food restaurant. Forty-five kids developed hemolytic uremic syndrome; three died. That was the tipping point. That, and the fact that Bill Clinton, the first baby boomer president of the United States, took office in January 1993. During his tenure, the entire food safety inspection system in the United States was revamped and Clinton made food safety one of his top priorities. The bacteria were not impressed. It is true that the massive investments in food safety during this time decreased the number of some foodborne illnesses in the 1990s, but those rates seem to have stabilized. Diseases related to *E. coli,* in particular, have not changed much. Bacteria can reorganize faster than people can.

In 1996, more than nine thousand children in Japan got sick when the white radish sprouts in their boxed lunches were contaminated. Twelve of them died.

Bacteria like *E. coli* are not the only waterborne microbes or even the most important ones, depending on how one judges importance. Other waterborne infections include the parasitic diseases cryptosporidiosis, caused by a single-celled organism that isn't bothered by chlorination, that is hard to find, and whose multiple homes and pathways into our drinking water researchers are only now beginning to unravel. And then there are the viruses.

In Florida, in 1986, after eating green salads at a floating restaurant, 103 people came down with hepatitis A, sometimes called infectious hepatitis or jaundice, an often-chronic debilitating viral disease that attacks your liver. In that case, the outbreak was traced to the less-than-clean food-handling habits of one of the bar employees, who helped tear up the salads (and also fix mixed drinks, another incriminated food). An epidemic of the same disease struck over a hundred people in Kentucky in 1988. That epidemic was linked to fresh iceberg lettuce, probably from Mexico. Also in 1988, more than three hundred *thousand* people, mostly between twenty and forty years old, came down with hepatitis in Shanghai; that outbreak was from infected shellfish, a perilous food, which I'll come back to in my zombies chapter. In 1997, almost three hundred school kids in the United States got hepatitis when they were served infected strawberries at school. The strawberries were supposed to be from California but were probably from Mexico or perhaps picked in the United States by underpaid Mexican workers who were not provided with good toilets, good pay, health insurance—all the amenities that are decent common sense to anyone but the "entrepreneurs" who own these places.

The most common group of foodborne viruses in North America, and probably the most common cause of foodborne or waterborne gut problems, are the Norwalk-like viruses, more recently given the official genus name norovirus. The first identified outbreak churned up the guts of a group of elementary school children in Norwalk, Ohio, in 1968. Four years later, an intrepid investigator fed stool filtrates (eau de poop?) from the original outbreak to volunteers. (Prisoners? Summer students? The report doesn't say.) The volunteers succumbed to nausea, vomiting, abdominal pain, diarrhea, low-grade fever, chills, malaise, anorexia, and headaches. I hope the volunteers were paid well or at least received good grades. Vomiting occurs more often in outbreaks involving children, and diarrhea more often in adults.

Since that first outbreak, scientists have discovered other viruses of the same family with names like Hawaii, MC, W, Ditchling, Cockle, Paramatta, Marin County, and Snow Mountain agents. As with most viruses, we get them either directly from other people or (perish the thought) through water that the viruses have, in polite terms, contaminated, and by so doing have found their way into clams, oysters, cockles, green salads, pastry, and frosting.

Sometimes reporters will announce that investigators are trying to determine whether an outbreak was foodborne or caused by noroviruses. This is a false dichotomy. Just because a disease-causing agent comes out of a person's bum doesn't mean it can't be foodborne. And just because it is foodborne doesn't mean it can't also get around in the water, on your hands, on the computer keys, and on doorknobs. It is possible to ride the bus and drive a car and ride a bicycle all in the same lifetime.

Finally, no discussion of waterborne diseases would be complete without looking at the mother of all of them: cholera. This waterborne disease, one of the classic diseases of socio-economic underdevelopment, has been well studied the world over. It has been endemic in eastern India and Bangladesh for thousands of years. From there, between 1817 and 1961, it spread around the world in seven major pandemics, killing millions of people regardless of race, creed, or color.

During the pandemic that passed through London from 1848 to 1854, John Snow, physician to Queen Victoria, carried out a series of now-famous epidemiological investigations, which demonstrated that people whose water was piped in by a particular company were about nine times more likely to die than people in the same neighborhood serviced by another company. The incriminated company drew its water from an especially polluted part of the Thames River. Both scientist and activist, Snow disabled the suspected Broad Street pump and studied the effects of his action on the incidence of cholera. In this way, some thirty-five years before Koch identified the offending organism, Snow was able to identify the vehicle of infection and the government was able to institute appropriate public health measures.

The seventh pandemic of cholera spread from Sulawesi, Indonesia, starting in 1961, and did not reach the Middle East,

Europe, and Africa until 1970. In 1991, it suddenly appeared in South America, where, taking advantage of crowding and poor sanitation in the huge shantytowns of cities such as Lima, Peru, it has demonstrated the natural consequences of global economic policies with a vengeance. One theory is that it arrived in the ballast of ships from the Far East. American scientist Rita Colwell has put forth compelling evidence to support a more complex and interesting story. Cholera organisms appear to be able to live in a dormant state along with algae or zooplankton (tiny sea animals). When the ocean is warm enough and is fortified with sufficient nutrients, the bacteria start multiplying. Global warming and nutrient runoff (think fertilizer and raw sewage, dumped into the oceans under the misconception that the ability of the oceans to dilute pollution is infinite) help create those perfect environments. Whatever the cause, it is fairly certain that we had a hand in creating those environments. In just a few years after 1991, tens of thousands of people became sick and hundreds died. El Tor, the strain of *Vibrio cholera* involved in the current pandemic, was named for a quarantine station in Egypt, where similar organisms were identified in 1886.

The vibrios cause disease by clinging to the intestinal walls, multiplying, and stimulating the body to secrete large amounts of fluids. In serious cases, profuse, watery diarrhea (rice-water stools) leads to dehydration (thirst, collapse, wrinkled skin, sunken eyes). Fever may occur in children. The ratio of severe to mild or asymptomatic cases has been estimated at 1:5 to 1:10 for classical cholera and 1:25 to 1:100 for El Tor. The most effective treatment is to stay hydrated with clean water containing a bit of salt, baking soda and sugar. But in the barrio, who has clean water?

During the South American epidemic, much of the spread was attributed to ceviche, a marinated fish dish. I have seen ceviche sold from the tailgates of trucks and seen the dirty water that can go into making it. For a few years, I refused to eat this raw fish gourmet delight, until a good Peruvian friend of mine persuaded me that I couldn't leave his country before having some. The setting for this suicidal act was a romantic restaurant in Lima. In the midafternoon, we looked out over the warm plaza, lovers strolling past, and I tasted my first tangy ceviche. I didn't get sick. In fact, it was wonderful, which says something about risks worth taking, which I shall come back to in a later chapter. The most nauseating part of the experience was a couple at a nearby table; she was talking into a cell phone, as was he, while the ambient bacteria dined on the romantic meal on the table between them.

Although *Vibrio cholera* is probably maintained in marine environments, once it gets into human society, it generally perpetuates itself through a cycle of infection in people, contamination of the environment, and re-infection of people. The vehicle of infection is almost always water contaminated with human feces or sewage. An outbreak in Jerusalem in 1970, for example, has been attributed by some authors to vegetables that were irrigated with waste water contaminated with human feces. In the South Pacific and in South America, water-contaminated dishes that include raw, salted fish are almost always to blame.

An organism from the same family, *Vibrio parahemolyticus*, was first associated with diarrheal disease in 1951, when almost three hundred people got sick and twenty died after eating *shirasu* (boiled and semidried young sardines) in Osaka, Japan. It was only after two other outbreaks that the organism was described and classified. One of these, involving salted cucumber, put 120 people into a Yokohama hospital in 1956; the other, traced to horse mackerel, affected thousands of Japanese along their Pacific coasts in 1960. The Japanese have become dramatically aware of the disease; about 0.5 percent of the total population is estimated to be infected during the summer months, and up to 50 percent of all cases of diarrheal food poisoning in summer are attributed to the organism.

V. parahemolyticus is now known to occur as well in many parts of South and East Asia, Europe, and the United States. It is not often reported in Canada, perhaps because of the cold coastal waters (which are warming up as a result of global warming, however). Crab, shrimp, lobster, and marine fish are the most common food vehicles. In the United States, the implicated food is often cooked and then recontaminated; in Japan, the vehicle is often a raw food. The organism is rarely found in deep-sea fish.

In both Japan and the United States, the disease is reported most often between June and October. If its cholera-producing sibling, like the dog, prefers the company of people, this one, catlike, ranges more freely. It can be isolated from sediment, plankton, sea fish, crustacea, and shellfish in coastal and estuarine environments.

A third member of this family, *Vibrio vulnificans,* has only been a public health concern for the last few decades. This organism is part of the normal marine flora and, using raw oysters as the ticket to get in, attacks men over forty years of age already debilitated by the likes of chronic liver disease, diabetes mellitus, various forms of cancer, and AIDS. Unlike the other vibrios, and perhaps because of the already poor health of its victims, this bug kills 40 to 60 percent of those it infects.

The vibrios are always a concern where poverty and natural disasters meet. After Hurricane Katrina hit New Orleans in 2005, for instance, twenty-two people got sick and five people died from illnesses cause by vibrios.

Waterborne infections, maybe more than most others, force us to face up to issues of ecological management and social justice. Washing your hands, well, that just doesn't quite cut it when there's sewage in the water, does it?

5

THE
YOUNG
AND THE
RETCHING

FOODBORNE BACTERIAL
INTOXICATIONS (EXCEPT BOTULISM)

"**THE YOUNG AND THE RETCHING**" was the title of a video created by some of my students as a class assignment. They figured it was the best way to communicate certain food safety messages to people who watched soap operas. The video told the story of a two-timing doctor, his wife, and their maid, who used *Staphylococcus aureus* to poison her rival, Mrs. Twotime. Colorless, odorless, and tasteless, staphylococcal toxin, which causes convulsive vomiting, was the perfect nonlethal weapon. Although the organisms are easily killed, the toxin itself can withstand boiling, irradiation, and the brutal buffeting of stomach acids. Thus, long after the organisms themselves are gone, they can wreak their havoc. And the toxin is readily available. *Staph* organisms are found on or in the skin, nose, hair, throat, and stool of 50 percent or more of the population in normal people and animals, and can also be procured from infected cuts and scabs in humans and animals and from the udders of infected cows. *Staph* organisms can persist in the digestive tracts of flies for several days.

So it should not be a surprise that staphylococcal food poisoning is one of the three or four most common types of food poisoning in North America and, indeed, the world. A 2002 study in the United States found that a quarter of outbreaks in schools for which the cause could be identified were caused by *Staph*. In some ways, it is because it is so common that we hear so little about it in the news. And because it is so common, it is not a legally reportable disease.

The diseases discussed in previous chapters are not, strictly speaking, food poisoning. They are infections, which require that bacteria grow in the food some time before they get to you and then multiply further in your body to produce some unwelcome outcome, often diarrhea. This process often takes a day or more, and sometimes much longer. Intoxication, or true food poisoning, occurs when the poison is in the food, you eat it, and then you get sick. For most toxins in our food, that sickness happens pretty quickly, within minutes or hours, as soon as the toxin hits those nerves that stimulate the brain's vomiting center. In this chapter and the next, I will focus on toxins produced by bacteria, rather than metals or industrial chemicals, which tend to have chronic effects and have quite a different ecology.

Staphylococcal food poisoning is caused by the toxins produced by the organism *Staphylococcus aureus*, or *Staph*, as it is often referred to in hallway conversations among food scientists and medical types. You can imagine the tiresome, endless punning possibilities: "Hey, did that *Staph* meeting yesterday ever make me sick." Or someone making throwing up noises in the bathroom, "I think the kitchen is over-*Staph*ed."

In the early part of the twenty-first century, disease care providers have most often expressed worries about methicillin-resistant *Staph aureus,* or MRSA, an organism that is resistant to our most common antibiotics. Sadly, MRSA seems to flourish in the places where we least want it—hospitals and nursing homes. By 1997, half of the *Staph* isolates in nursing homes and hospitals in the United States were MRSA.

For a long time, however, public health workers didn't worry about it as a foodborne organism. Then, in 2002, three people came down with nausea, vomiting, and cramps a few hours after eating shredded barbecued pork and coleslaw from a local delicatessen. Investigators found *Staph* all over the place, but the outbreak strain seemed to come from one particular food preparer, who had visited an aging relative in a nursing home who had died from a staphylococcal infection.

Although MRSA has been uncommon in community-based outbreaks, *Staph aureus* in general has been, and remains, a major cause of food poisoning worldwide. People in hospitals may have higher rates of carrying the bug than other people, but it is, one might say, ubiquitous, which, not accidentally, I would say, rhymes with "iniquitous," which is another way of saying that this bug is wickedly everywhere.

Staph toxins were first related to disease in 1914, when M.A. Barber demonstrated that people got sick from drinking unrefrigerated milk from a cow with mastitis. This relationship was forgotten and rediscovered in 1929, when human volunteers (the nature of whom I have been unable to determine—nonunionized lab assistants?), were fed cream-filled sponge cakes containing *Staph* toxins. Within a few hours of eating, they all became ill with nausea, vomiting, retching, abdominal pain, diarrhea, and prostration. Since then, people eating high-protein cooked foods conform to the usual risk profile for *Staph* sufferers. One typical example, taken from my files, is titled:

"Staphylococcal food poisoning on a cruise ship." It begins with the lines, "Two waves of vomiting and/or diarrhea affected approximately 215 of the 715 passengers on a Caribbean cruise ship. The outbreak was independently associated with eating cream-filled pastries..."

Since the organisms love precooked foods of high protein content, North American eating habits place us at risk for this intoxication. Foods like ham, meat and poultry products, cream, and cheese are often the vehicle for intoxication. In Japan, rice balls, prepared by hand and unrefrigerated, are a common vehicle. We tend to think of *Staph* food poisoning as occurring in small outbreaks, but the times, as Bob Dylan once said, are a-changing. Like other foodborne diseases, *Staph* outbreaks are getting larger, more geographically spread out, or both.

In 1989, outbreaks of staphylococcal food poisoning in the United States were traced to canned mushrooms from the People's Republic of China. The source of the outbreaks was a puzzle. *Staph* organisms do not usually compete well with the millions of other bacteria that grow on mushrooms; the mushrooms would be reduced to mush by spoilage bacteria before the *Staph* had managed to drum up enough poison to make anyone seriously puke. It also seemed unlikely that the poison had gotten into the cans after the mushrooms had been canned. Nature's Farm Products, Inc., of California, a top importer of mushrooms from China into the United States, put together a team of scientists to investigate this mystery. What they came up with should serve as a cautionary tale for all of us.

High-quality canning mushrooms are grown on collectives in Fujian, China, during the cool season, from November to March. No refrigeration is then necessary for the usual 30- to 50-mile trip to the canning factory. Picked each morning and trucked in polyethylene crates to the local plant, the mushrooms are inspected, graded, blanched, sized, sliced, and packed into tins, which are then sealed, steamed, and re-inspected two weeks later. Most of the work in these plants is done by hand, so the mushrooms could be contaminated, but the organisms would not have time to grow before they were destroyed by heat.

No obvious flaws in the system presented themselves to the scientists. They then took a slight step back, to get a wider view of the situation. During 1989, as the Chinese government encouraged private initiative, mushrooms became a valuable free-market commodity. Speculators from Hong Kong began buying mushrooms from the Fujian collectives, and the local packing plants had to seek supplies farther afield. Now, instead of getting mushrooms in two to four hours from growers they knew, plants received their goods in 44-pound polyethylene bags several days after the growers had harvested the mushrooms.

Mushrooms use up a lot of oxygen in a short amount of time. The researchers calculated that the mushrooms in the plastic bags would quickly use up their available oxygen supply, and the levels of carbon dioxide would rise correspondingly. The carbon dioxide, in turn, would, like an authoritarian state, drive the air-loving spoilage bacteria into quiescence, allowing the toxin-producing *Staph* to outcompete them. The mushrooms would arrive at the plant looking okay but full enough of poison to make a stir-fry into a stomach-churn.

The scientists tried to reproduce these conditions experimentally by putting mushrooms into plastic bags, throwing in some *Staph* organisms, and checking in on them after a couple of days. Not only did the bugs grow and make toxins as the scientists had suspected, but bags with only the normal environmental populations of bacteria and no extra *Staph* thrown in also produced the toxins.

In 1998, eight thousand folks gathered to celebrate the ordination of a priest in Minas Gerais, Brazil, either because they liked him a lot or because free chicken, roast beef, rice, and beans were being served. The eight food handlers started getting everything ready on Friday and kept everything in aluminum containers until it was needed on Sunday. Within four hours of eating, four thousand of the celebrants were bent over with vomiting, pain, diarrhea, and dizziness. About two thousand people needed medical attention, and almost four hundred were admitted to hospital, eighty-one of them into intensive care; sixteen people—all either over sixty-five or younger than five—died. Although these events might give Catholics reason to ponder what sort of a god would inflict this on his people, they should take heart that they are not alone: this food-poisoning god is generous in bestowing his afflictions.

In late June and early July 2000, in Japan, while everyone was heaving a sigh of relief that the millennium computer "bug" hadn't brought down the world's computers and hence ended all modern life on the planet, more than thirteen thousand people got sick from eating powdered skim milk, contaminated with *Staph* toxin.

Staphylococcus aureus isn't the only common organism to produce toxins. On a Monday evening in August 2003, five Belgian children were served some leftover pasta. The pasta had been prepared Friday for a picnic on Saturday. The leftovers were kept in the refrigerator. A fourteen-year-old boy and two girls, one ten and one nine, didn't eat much. They thought the food smelled bad. A dutiful seven-year-old girl and a nine-year-old boy apparently ate what was put before them. The youngest girl started vomiting six hours later; she had trouble breathing and was taken to the hospital. By the time they got there, everybody was throwing up. The youngest girl and the nine-year-old boy were getting worse quickly and had to be intubated. The youngest girl went into a coma, bleeding into her lungs, and died from acute liver failure thirteen hours after her meal. The nine-year-old boy was kept on a ventilator and given fluids and survived, but barely.

These children suffered from a severe form of foodborne intoxication, caused by a bacterium called *Bacillus cereus*, which affects hundreds of North Americans at a minimum, and uncounted people in other cultures, every year. In the 1960s, it was the third most common form of food poisoning in Hungary, associated with well-spiced meat dishes; spores from the organism were found in some of the spices used.

Vomiting disease caused by *B. cereus* is sometimes thought of as a kind of "Chinese restaurant" syndrome, because it is commonly found in rice paddies and is well adapted to some of the ways rice is prepared. If one were such a bacillus, one might wish for a heaven where rice is prepared ahead of time and then stored in the kitchen until used, perhaps even a day later: the initial cooking kills the mother cells but leaves spores behind. In this Nirvana, leftovers are commonly kept around (allowing the spores to start reproducing like mad, which is what bacteria love best), and guilt and not eating what's on your plate are kissing cousins (allowing people to ingest the bacteria and their toxins). As a bacterium, one might even thrill at the thought of surviving a quick flash-fry just before reincarnation in another human body.

The Chinese restaurant syndrome makes a neat story but is a bit misleading, as the pasta episode made clear. And that was not an isolated case (although its seriousness was unusual). An outbreak at a wedding reception reported in 2006 from Salerno, Italy, was traced to ricotta cheese. In 2002, in Quebec, partygoers got sick from contaminated mayonnaise used to make potato salad. At a "handicapped sports day" in Thailand, half of more than a thousand people were challenged with both *B. cereus* and *Staph aureus*; éclairs were the culprit that time. *B. cereus* has been found in probiotics used to prevent disease and has even caused scalp infections in new military recruits in Georgia; bad haircuts were blamed for that outbreak. Because the organism is so widespread and holidays just about everywhere, it seems to cause problems wherever food is abused.

If we try to kill *Bacillus* organisms by cooking, they leave behind spores. The spores survive boiling and frying; if we then leave the food at room temperature for a while, vegetative growth is rapid. It doesn't even mind mild refrigeration; the pasta that caused the Belgian family such anguish was stored in a refrigerator at about 57°F. A really good refrigerator, the kind a wealthy family might own, should take your food down to about 39°F.

B. cereus also makes a toxin that causes diarrhea and that has effects similar to those caused by *Clostridium perfringens*, another of those organisms found in the environment, as well as in human stools and food, and that is associated, under very different circumstances, with both gas gangrene and diarrhea. When large numbers of *C. perfringens* are eaten (remember what I said earlier about its reproductive prowess?), they wait until they get into the human intestine before generating spores (sporulating) and producing toxin. Like the *C. perfringens* toxin, the *B. cereus* diarrhea toxin is produced mostly in the intestine, so the disease occurs about ten to twelve hours after eating (rather than five or six), and thus is not, strictly speaking, an intoxication. Unlike *C. perfringens*, *B. cereus* does produce some toxin in the food. This toxin, however, is a lot less stable than its vomiting partner and is destroyed by most common cooking procedures. The emetic (vomit-causing) toxin, by contrast, can withstand heating at 250°F for an hour and can also survive some pretty strong acids and bases. Fortunately, the diarrhea-and-cramps form is both less stable and produces less severe disease than the vomiting form.

Bacillus cereus comes from a nasty family. With the advent of newer molecular techniques and the ability to examine genetic material more precisely, we now think that *B. cereus sensu stricto* (that is, *B. cereus* in the strictest sense of the term) is the same species as *B. thuringiensus* and *B. anthracis*. All belong to

B. cereus sensu lato—that is, *B. cereus* in the broad sense—and occupy similar, and occasionally the same, ecological niches in the soil.

Those of you who read the newspapers or, better yet, who have read my book on zoonoses, will recognize *B. anthracis* as the bug that causes anthrax. Environmentalists might recognize the *B. thuringiensus* as an organism that is known to infect insects and that has been used as a natural pesticide to control mosquitoes in areas where malaria and dengue fever are common. One might wonder if this might be a little like relying on Hell's Angels to provide security at a rock concert. If the bacteria behave well, keep their behavior in their genes, and focus on keeping mosquitoes in line, the practice just might work. But in biology, as in rock concerts, things are never quite that stable. *B. thuringiensus* grows well in the guts of a variety of insects and invertebrates, such as earthworms, and does not necessarily kill them. These creatures may spread the organisms, which may kill or devour their hosts only if they are weakened or die from other causes. Like *B. thuringiensus*, *B.cereus sensu stricto*, the bacterium we associate with foodborne illness, probably lives its normal, natural life in the guts of soil-dwelling insects and probably in a filamentous, plantlike form. *B. cereus* has been found in human fecal samples at rates of anywhere from 10 to more than 40 percent. Being so widespread in our food supplies, they are mostly just tourists passing through the much celebrated (in the bacterial world) tunnel of love, our mammalian intestines. Like most bacteria, they only cause trouble if we encourage them.

C. perfringens and *B. cereus* remind us, once again, that we are part of a large, sprawling, brawling ecological family and that we know almost nothing about even our closest relatives. They are small visitors from our country cousins who live in the soil, who want to remind us where we come from, who, if we abuse them, are not averse to taking revenge. The message of *Staph aureus* is both a little more pedestrian (wash your hands before preparing food, and, if you feel a sneeze coming on, stick your nose into the pit of your elbow, not your hand) and a little more political (changes in economic policies in China can sabotage a romantic stir-fry in California).

6

GRANDMA'S
REVENGE

BOTULISM

W HAT DO THE Sibo minority in China,
New York Jews, circumpolar Inuit, Vancouver yuppies, Georgian peasants, and
German sausage eaters have in common? Oh, and as of 2006,
carrot juice drinkers? This could be the beginning of a really
bad joke. The title of this chapter is the punch line.

In mid-July 1985, an Inuit hunter near Lake Harbour, Northwest Territories, killed and gutted a walrus; the following day,
pieces of walrus meat, fat, and bone were put into two skin
pouches, tied shut, and hung in the open air, in direct sunlight, for two weeks. At the end of that month, eleven adults
and one child in Lake Harbour ate this fermented walrus meat,
along with cooked caribou, fish, raw and dried seal meat, eggs,
and beef. Within twenty-four hours, one twenty-nine-year-old

woman complained of nausea, vomiting, blurred vision, and a dry mouth. Some of her friends also did not feel well. Fortunately, all were given botulinum antitoxin and no one died.

In June 2002, a dead adult beluga washed up on the shores of the Bering Sea near a fishing village in western Alaska. Several weeks later, the villagers stumbled across this gift from the gods and harvested skin and pink blubber from the fluke (tail) to make muktuk. It was stored in zipper-sealed plastic bags in a refrigerator. A couple of days later, fourteen people shared the feast. Eight of them came down with botulism. Two of them had to be put onto mechanical ventilators until their bodies had processed the toxin. All of them, fortunately, survived. About a year earlier, across the border in northern British Columbia, a seventy-three-year-old mother and her fifty-year-old son finished off a jar of fermented salmon roe; the next day, they both needed respirators. The mother had a heart attack and died.

The rate of botulism in native people in northern Canada and Alaska is consistently several thousand times as high as that of the non-native population. Among those who get it, a lot more native people die, although this situation is improving. Why such a high rate? In native people, most cases are associated with traditional Inuit foods (such as *urraq*—seal flippers in oil; *muktuk*—whale blubber with skin and meat; and *micerak*—seal, whale, or walrus fat), as well as with fermented salmon eggs, eaten by Pacific Northwest native groups.

Fermented seafoods are somewhat risky business at the best of times. They contain little carbohydrate, which is necessary to produce acid quickly and hence inhibit the organisms that cause the disease. Moreover, native people are sometimes understandably hesitant to go to a medical clinic—if there is a medical clinic available—for fear of hearing another lecture on the dangers of native foods. Often they arrive too late to get the lifesaving antitoxin, or they have severe breathing problems and cannot get to a respirator (often an airplane trip away) to keep them alive until the poison wears off. Since the first edition of this book came out, the death rate, at least, has been declining, meaning that people are getting treatment sooner. Case fatality rates (the number of deaths among those who get sick) in Canada dropped from 45 percent in the 1960s to less than 3 percent in the 1990s.

Botulism toxin has been called the most potent toxin known to man. Or is it dioxin? Or aflatoxin? I get confused sometimes. I suppose the classification of toxins depends in part on your politics. With botulism, for instance, the phrase "to man" might be a key. Some men might see it as being the most potent toxin because they are dependent on a woman's practice of the mysterious art of cooking; she could slip the stuff into your food. You start to feel tingly and a little weak-kneed, and you think that this food is fine and the woman is being nice to you. Then you see double (too much wine), you have trouble speaking, and there's a tightness at your throat (gosh, I think I'm in love). It is only when the weakness in your body grips you around the rib cage and you stop breathing that you think: botulism. This is the sort of misogynist male paranoia out of which you could make a movie, or you could use it as part of your anti-political-correctness-I-know-what's-best-for-you political campaign. Many of my students have seen a movie like this. It is never a comedy.

For those of us who know a little bit about food, cooking, and the environment—who are aware, that is, of who we are and where we live and have some basic life skills—botulism is no great mystery. The organism that produces the toxin, *Clostridium botulinum,* is a member of a family of bacteria, including *C. perfringens,* mentioned in the previous chapter, that lives just about everywhere. *C. botulinum* prefers an environment that is not acidic (which is why it likes carrots better than tomatoes) and that has no oxygen (conditions found in foil-wrapped

potatoes, garlic in oil, and canned ham and canned beans). It
has been found in soils at glacial heights of more than 9,800 feet
and down to a thousand fathoms in the sea. C. *botulinum* produces spores that survive boiling and irradiation and will germinate if the food is left at room temperature long enough. This
is why you need to can beans in a pressure cooker—to crank
the temperature up over 212°F. So the organisms are often in
our food. The toxin, unlike that of C. *perfringens,* is produced
only in the food (infant botulism being an exception, which I
shall come around to a bit later), and only when the organisms
are deprived of oxygen. Fortunately, botulinum toxin itself is
destroyed easily by cooking (boiling a few minutes or cooking at
more than 185°F for a bit longer).

The word "botulinum" comes from the Latin for sausage,
and with good reason. In Germany, where the Western understanding of the disease comes from, it was historically associated with eating spoiled sausage. One author, Justin Kerner,
who wrote in the early 1800s about what was then called Kerner's disease, described 230 instances of this sausage poisoning.
It was not until 1897, when twenty-three of thirty-four members
of a German musical band playing a funeral gig got into some
spoiled ham, that the organisms and toxins were identified.

As a child, I was advised to avoid eating from jars of canned
beans in which the lid had buckled upwards, because the buck-
ling indicated that bacteria inside were producing gas (a good
laugh for a teenager). Back then, people lumped together most
foodborne illnesses into something called ptomaine poisoning,
believed to be caused by consuming the bacterial products of
putrefaction. Larry's mother, in Carol Shields' novel *Larry's Party,*
accidentally killed her mother-in-law with botulism by feeding
her poorly canned beans. That was the sort of thing my mother
worried about. I do not recall her ever saying anything about
fermented whale blubber or garlic in oil (which were pretty

far outside our usual Mennonite fare) or even sausages, with which my Dad occasionally got paid for preaching in small country churches.

In the early part of this century, most cases of botulism could be traced to improper canning procedures, first, of commercial foods, and then, after these were regulated (in the 1920s), home-canned foods. After that, most of the world took canned goods for granted. Then, in the country formerly known as the Soviet Republic of Georgia, now just Georgia, things fell apart. From the 1980s to the late 1990s, the rate of botulism in Georgia tripled, at which time it had the highest rate of any country in the world. Most of the cases were related to home-canned vegetables. Like the people of the North, the Georgians had forgotten the lessons of their grandmothers.

Because *C. botulinum* is found all over the world, botulism is a great cross-cultural leveler. After chuckling over the culinary weirdnesses of those northern Inuit, people in other parts of the world may themselves start to feel weak.

Kapchunka (also called ribbetz) is a salted, air-dried whitefish beloved of many people of Eastern European descent. In October 1987, a gentleman purchased two ribbetz from a Brooklyn delicatessen as a gift to take back to Israel to his wife and his brother's family. His wife was pleased and, in celebration, ate seven ounces or so of the whitefish. Twelve hours later, she was in respiratory intensive care with double vision, slurred speech, vomiting, and progressive weakness of her extremities. She also had difficulty breathing. In another twelve hours, her mother was admitted to hospital with a tentative diagnosis of congestive heart failure. Not until after the mother had died, five hours after admission, did Jerusalem health district officers begin putting the picture together. The full investigation turned up eight cases of botulism, six in Israel and two in New York, all traced to ribbetz bought at the same deli.

Women of the Sibo ethnic group in China, in preparing a special sauce for their April festival, steamed pieces of bread, placed them in a pot under several layers of cloth, and let them ferment for a few weeks. It is the kind of thing you have to nibble at to make sure it is doing okay. As a result, every year women and children among the Sibo suffered a mysterious neurological ailment that peaked in April. When the bread was done, it was powdered and mixed with boiling water, thus neutralizing the toxin before the men got at it.

In March 2006, more than 150 people came down with botulism in Thailand, after eating pickled bamboo shoots at a Buddhist festival. They had to fly in antitoxin from Canada, the United States, the United Kingdom, and Japan.

Nineteen eighty-five was also a bad year for a couple of Vancouver restaurants. One of them, a popular fast food place near Stanley Park, unwittingly served contaminated chopped garlic in soybean oil in a couple of their sandwiches. Because of the nature of the restaurant, and the small amounts of garlic eaten, people as far away as the Netherlands and parts of the United States were, in the weeks that followed, hospitalized with a range of neurologic and psychiatric disorders.

A second, classier restaurant served their special in-house chanterelle mushrooms as part of a delectable and no doubt expensive dish called Fricassée de Rouget-Barbet and Lobster with Wild Mushrooms. The mushrooms were wild all right: of thirty-one people who dined on this delicacy, six had tingling and numbness, five of them ending up in the hospital, three of those five on respirators.

Today three main types of botulism are seen in North America. The first, called wound botulism, I won't cover here, but it is associated with deep wounds. The second form is the adult foodborne botulism; although this form is still sometimes associated with home-canned foods in Europe and North America, most attention has been shifted to the "usual" outbreaks resulting from garlic in oil, foil-wrapped potatoes, carrot juice, and fermented seafoods. A third kind of botulism, infant botulism, deserves at least a passing mention, if only because it is the most common form of botulism reported in the United States.

First diagnosed in 1931 in a three-month-old infant in California, infant botulism was essentially not reported again until the mid-1970s. About a hundred cases per year are diagnosed in the United States; about half of these occur in California. In Canada cases are rare (seven cases in twenty-five years). These patterns of occurrence have never been satisfactorily explained, to me at least. It has been suggested that infant botulism is one cause of sudden infant death syndrome.

Babies with infant botulism become constipated, lose head control, and sometimes die. This kind of botulism is unusual because it occurs in the absence of preformed toxin ingestion. It is suggested that clostridial spores are eaten and that they germinate and multiply in the child's intestine and produce toxin. The absence of competitive flora may explain why this happens in infants and not in adults.

Mothers of babies who have infant botulism are reported to be better educated and to breast-feed more than mothers of babies who don't get the disease, but one might wonder if this discrepancy has to do with access to good diagnostic acumen and good health care or to the fact that babies of less-educated mothers die of other causes. About 15 percent of the cases have been attributed to honey contaminated with botulinum spores. *C. botulinum* may be more common in the soils in areas where the disease is more common. In most countries of the world that have poor health care and lots of ways for babies to die, this form of botulism probably occurs but is not reported.

Having said so much that is negative about the botulinum neurotoxin, I feel constrained to balance the picture a little. Botulinum toxin's therapeutic uses include, according to one review, "the correction of focal dystonias and other regional movement disorders." A layperson might understandably imagine these to have something to do with the correction of musical (dystonia) and military (regional movements) disorders; in fact, in going over the list of clinical signs that this powerful toxin has been used to alleviate, I see "musician's cramp" and "uncontrollable anal sphincter contraction"—so the lay interpretation may not be so far off after all. The basis of these therapeutic uses is that the toxin blocks the release of a major neurotransmitter (acetylcholine) and thereby encourages relaxation. If you can target it so that your breathing muscles do not get too relaxed, it can thus be used to relieve some forms of muscular cramping. Lest anyone forget that we are talking about one of the most potent toxins on the planet, however, I hasten to add that I know at least one person who almost died when the doctor got sloppy and accidentally injected the toxin into a blood vessel. One variation of the toxin, botox, is also used for getting rid of wrinkles and laugh lines—you know, those things on our faces that make us look human.

The tales of gastrointestinal woe associated with variations of Grandma's cooking are endless, but botulism, to me, covers most of the finger-wagging ground. Some, probably many, of the foodborne epidemics that now blow through the global food system are the result of some combination of the loss of traditional cooking skills and maladaptation in a social, economic, and environmental context that is very different from the ones in which they were devised.

The farther we get away from our ancestral homes, the rustier we become. In my home, recipes were never written down. Mother told my older sister how to make things, but I, as a struggling male novice at the kitchen counter, have to make do with what has been scribbled into the folds of my failing cerebral cortex. Traditional foods may thus be improperly prepared, magnifying an inherent risk. Whereas traditionally fermented Inuit foods were put into covered pits in the permafrost, where they underwent a slow, cool fermentation, the modern cooks want to speed things up. They put the flippers or blubber into plastic bags or buckets and hang them on the washline or set them out on the porch; in spring and summer, the temperature might just be close enough to bacterial heaven to approximate gastronomical hell. Global warming just makes it all worse. The high incidence of botulism among the Inuit may reflect a loss of traditional knowledge in combination with a changing climate.

Mimicking Grandma but not having properly learned her skills, and not knowing why she did what she did (if she had a reason), we suffer her revenge: Thought I was old-fashioned, did ya? Thought you could improve on my cooking, eh?

7

IT MAY BE WORMS TO YOU (BUT IT'S MY BREAD AND BUTTER)

PARASITES

W HEN I ARRIVED in Kathmandu, Nepal, in 1991, livestock were slaughtered along the banks of the Bishnumati River. In the predawn, buffaloes were pithed with a hammer and spike. Straw was piled over them and set on fire to burn off the hair. There in the dirt, the animals were gutted, skinned, and prepared for the meat market. Dogs and pigs wandered about, scavenging what they could get. A variety of species, including people, defecated at the water's edge, where others were washing utensils. *Echinococcus granulosus,* a tapeworm in dogs that forms tumorlike hydatid cysts in the livers and lungs of livestock and people, was but one of many issues with which the Nepalese people had to deal. When I came back home to Canada, I confess I lent a less-than-sympathetic ear to complaints about our lot, the cost of food, the cost of fuel, all that stuff. In the years since I first visited that area of Kathmandu, the situation is much improved, in part, I would like to think, because of some of my interventions.

Since then, as well, it has become increasingly clear that parasitic contamination of food in North America and Europe is more common than we like to think, enough so as to help a few parasitologists put dinner on the family table.

Taenia solium is a large, glistening, segmented tapeworm that lives as an adult in the intestines of humans. If we listen carefully, we may learn a great deal about politics, culture, nature, and religion from the voice of this parasite. The larva spends a protected childhood encapsulated in a cyst in the meat of pigs. These cysts were once referred to as cysticercus cellulosae, or the pork tapeworm, before their full life's tale had unfolded. Pigs, those voracious, fun-loving, hypochondriac omnivores so much like ourselves, become infected by eating human waste, offered to them through the careless recycling of sewage as fertilizer for field crops that are subsequently used as animal feed. In an ironic pact with nature, anyone who eats the meat of these infected pigs, whose bodies have been sacrificed for our pleasure, can suffer an intestinal affliction with the adult worm, thus completing this cycle of life. Occasionally, people may infect themselves, taking the role of the pig in the cycle, and the parasite may migrate to the brain, where it may be associated with epileptic convulsions and other neurological problems.

The Italian holocaust survivor Primo Levi wrote a strange and beautiful psalm of celebration using the voice of a tapeworm, ambiguously omitting the particular name of the worm. For a Jew or a Muslim, infection with *T. solium* could be seen as a natural-cum-religious consequence of transgressing the boundaries of appropriate human diet. One might even think of the brain infection variation as a kind of occult possession.

The churning in the intestines is thus a mirror of a more deeply felt spiritual tremor. In East Africa, the connection is not the result of carelessness and is more heart wrenching: poor villagers are given pigs so that they can raise money to send their children, and the dozens of AIDS orphans they have taken in, to school. Being poor, however, they don't have feed for the pigs, which scavenge what they can. This situation is compounded by the fact that proper latrines are not available and, physicians, who practice that subspecialty of veterinary medicine, naked primate medicine, are generally not aware of the connections between the parasite and epilepsy.

Levi might have been writing about *Taenia saginata,* a human tapeworm that comes back to us through beef. Although full of moral significance for Hindus, infections with this tapeworm would be morally neutral for Muslims and Jews. *T. saginata* is very rarely reported in people or animals in Canada. In cattle it is called *Cysticercus bovis.* In the United States, the rate detected in cattle at slaughter is higher than in Canada—about 20 per 100,000 cattle slaughtered. One Canadian exception to this general rule occurred in Ontario in 1993, when cattle from a certain feedlot were found to have an infection rate of more than 7 percent. The cattle may have acquired the tapeworm eggs from an infected, underpaid farm worker who did not have an outhouse readily available, or from vegetables grown on land irrigated with sewage sludge or otherwise contaminated. Indeed, the source, via infected farm workers, may have been somewhere in the southern United States or Mexico, where this infection in people is much more common.

In the United States, the rates of infection with *Cysticercus bovis* are twelve times as high in California as elsewhere. Immigrant workers—and cattle—from farther south, where the infection is common, as well as the use of recycled water and sewage effluent for irrigation and watering pastures, may be the cause of these increased rates.

Primo Levi might have seen another tapeworm as a celebration of his culinary heritage. Gefilte fish is a delicacy prepared from minced fish pressed into balls and boiled until done. As every good cook knows, the best way to tell if something is done is to taste it. In just this way, then, many a Jewish grandmother has invited into her bowels the larvae of *Diphyllobothrium latum.* These parasites thrive in that center of culinary culture, growing to great lengths to reproduce themselves, sending babies off into the wide, watery world to be properly schooled, if not thwarted by proper sewage disposal, in the fleshy ways of freshwater fish. Ultimately, they return to us to turn our stomachs and give us crawly bums. Jewish grandmothers are not the only ones who suffer for their children's good cuisine.

Nor are they the only ones who suffer for the sake of ethnically friendly fish cuisine. A wave of interest in raw fish prepared Japanese style has stimulated a wave of interest in several parasites that normally cycle between marine mammals and fish. *Phocanema decipiens* is a roundworm that normally migrates from seals, where it lives as an adult, through various species of fish, where it wriggles out a vigorous larval adolescence, and then makes its way back to the warm mammalian safety of the seal again. If an infected fish is not properly cleaned immediately after being caught, the larval worm may escape its offal home and camouflage itself in the whiteness of the fish flesh. Later, lurking as quietly and cunningly in a pickled herring as Delilah in her silken sheets, the worm may emerge, curious and persistent, using its boring tooth to dig through the human's stomach wall and go exploring in the dark, fleshy depths of this unfamiliar mammal. The resulting severe, sporadic stomach pain, nausea, and vomiting—if it is properly diagnosed—is called acute gastric anasikiasis, or sometimes, popularly, sushi worm.

Those affected find it far from boring. The only cure is surgery. Fortunately, it is a rare affliction, and the results are not normally quite so dramatic. According to Peter Schantz of the

Centers for Disease Control and Prevention, these worms are "usually coughed up or regurgitated . . . producing astonishment but no disease."

Most parasitic infections acquired from raw fish are reported from people preparing their food at home, rather than in those who dine out at sushi or sashimi restaurants. A survey of sushi restaurants in Seattle found that one in thirteen slices of sushi contained larvae, but the larvae were dead, indicating that the fish had probably been frozen before serving. The dead larvae are not a health risk, but I know at least one biologist who has used his ability to point out the dead larvae in his sushi to the waiter or waitress to obtain free food.

In our eating, we demonstrate also our separateness: what do we not eat? Jews have always been well aware of this separateness. Daniel and his young friends, captives of a foreign state, insisted on a vegetarian diet, I am convinced, not because the diet itself was any more righteous than that of the royal court, but because, like the wearing of Amish black hats, saffron-colored robes, or facial veils, it was a statement of belonging to a community different from the general culture. It was a statement of independence.

Trichinosis is a parasitic disease that cycles between carnivores. It is historically associated with a rat-pig-human-rat cycle, but more recently has been reported among bears, Inuit, organic gourmands, and French hunters. Because the disease is associated with pigs, its absence in Jews and Muslims sets them apart from many other religious or ethnic groups.

The first clinical case of trichinosis was recognized in Germany, during the Christmas season of 1859. A young servant girl, preparing meats for the holiday, felt dizzy and tired, and her muscles ached. Friedrich Albert von Zenker, a pathologist at the Dresden hospital, diagnosed her as having typhoid fever (a kind of salmonellosis passed from people to people, not involving other animals). The servant girl lay curled up in extreme pain and died fifteen days after entering the hospital. Zenker, wishing to confirm his original diagnosis, did a complete post-mortem, which included taking a sliver of her muscle, crushing it, and looking at it under the microscope; the muscle was wriggling with tiny worms.

As has happened often in the history of foodborne disease, once the disease was recognized, many more epidemics appeared, and it did not take long to connect the human disease with the tiny white flecks in pork. The life cycle of this parasite, which can infect any carnivore, is quite simple. Cysts containing larval parasites are eaten with the meat in which they are embedded. Once in your intestine, the parasites excyst (slip out of their cysts) and, attaching to the intestinal crypts, develop into adults in the space of several days, and copulate. Then—in a development that makes me glad that Solomon advised us to go to the ants rather than to the trichinae—the males are discarded. Over the next few weeks, the young larvae enter your bloodstream and are scattered throughout the body, eventually settling down in striated muscle, where they wait for you to encounter rats or cannibals. Historically, pigs have been identified as the major source of the disease for people of German, Italian, or Polish descent.

At the end of the nineteenth century, the Germans, having decided that worms were not to be tolerated in their summer sausage, established an army of 100,000 inspectors, with a budget greater than that of the United States Department of Agriculture, to test pigs at slaughterhouses. The Americans, however, only tested for it when the Germans made it a trade issue—and then only for the export market, not to protect their own consumers.

By the middle of the 1990s, North Americans thought we were largely rid of this disease. Changes from outdoor free-range management of swine to indoor confinement, regulation of garbage feeding, and tendencies to cook pork longer than other meats all helped to control the infection. Freezing destroys the form of the parasite found in southern swine, but not the northern form found in bears, wolves, foxes, and seals in Hudson's Bay. The disease persists in North America, as well as in Europe, where more than a thousand cases a year are still diagnosed. The human disease is seen especially among those who prefer free-running pigs that have had access to rats. About 2 percent of North American bears harbor the parasite and are a source of disease for those who live in or visit the Canadian North.

In the United States, the annual number of reported clinical cases dropped from almost five hundred in 1950 to one-tenth of that in 1985. The cases that do appear target certain ethnic groups. Although the infection rate in pigs is probably less than half a percent, less than half a percent of a hundred million hogs butchered every year in the United States is a lot of contaminated pork chops. In the United States, between 1975 and 1984, the incidence of reported clinical trichinosis (fever, aching muscles, and puffy eyes) was twenty-five times greater for Southeast Asian refugees—Laotians and Cambodians, in particular—than for the general U.S. population.

In the 1980s, some unusual outbreaks hit horse-meat eaters in France and Italy who consumed imports from the United States. How could the noncarnivorous horses get the little worms into their system? The European importers might suggest that ground-up rats infested the horse feed—to which the American exporters might respond that the French butchers had knives, saws, and cutting boards wriggling with the little creatures before the horses ever bit the bullet. Unfortunately for the Americans-are-pigs argument, there have been more than three thousand horse-meat-related cases of trichinosis in the European Union since the 1970s. Still, there is a niggling suspicion that many of these cases are from horses that acquired infection outside the EU.

The French got hit in the muscle again in 2005. On August 26, 2005, a hunting party from France killed a black bear in northern Quebec, Canada. They skinned the animal, eviscerated it, and cut it up for eating. Over the next week, they ate the bear meat in various forms and varying degrees of doneness, from fully cooked stews to a little taste of raw. They were, after all, citizens of the country that has given the world steak tartare. A couple of the hunters smuggled some meat back home in their luggage and had parties with their friends in France. When epidemiologists put together the finally tally, there were seventeen cases of trichinosis, all caused by the northern, freezer-friendly form of the parasite.

If a fascination with Canadian wilderness had an unexpected effect on French hunters, so too did a misplaced understanding of what "wild" and "organic" mean to a group of Ontario gourmand meat eaters. Indeed, one might imagine the worms anticipating at least one of these "specialty" meat sources with some excitement: "Running, running, his nose to the ground, the scratch of dry branches against his itchy hide. There, a warm smell, the smell of fear, of flesh, blood, the crunch of rat in his mouth. The good warm taste. That's us he's eating; that's us he's tasting. He doesn't know it, stupid old boar."

"We have been hiding in the nurse cells, muscle cells that we have specially modified to nurture us. When the cells are eaten, our little Trojan horses are digested away in the gut, and then our babies grow, and molt, and grow and molt. Four times. And then we are adults. Well, breeding age, is that adult? What a celebration! We breed like crazy, and the little babies wiggle their butts across the gut wall into the bloodstream. They are looking for muscle cells. Nurse cells. And then our babies will crouch inside, and wait. Our kind can wait for a long time. For years. Forever. Someone will shoot us. Someone will warm us over the fire. Someone will free us. We will breed, oh what a joy, we will breed."

But of course, people who eat meats like wild boar cannot imagine the lives of parasites; for not the first time, such an impoverishment of the imagination can be directly linked to disease. In January 1993, more than two dozen people throughout the Guelph, Kitchener and Toronto areas were diagnosed with trichinosis. The disease was traced to cold-smoked and dried sausage made from commercially grown wild boar meat and sold through farmers' markets. People who know wild boars better than I do tell me that these animals will eat anything— rats, mice, each other, tourists, farmers. They therefore have plenty of opportunity to pick up infections and parasites from wild animals. The meat was sold as organic and, by implication, both environmentally and physiologically friendly. Environmentally friendly and natural wild boars may be, but so are *Trichinella* parasites.

Many of the parasites in food that concern us can be avoided by cooking food well. Anywhere from a third to three-quarters of all adults in the world are infected with *Toxoplasma gondii*. The parasite is maintained by members of the cat family, and although it only causes aches and pains in nonpregnant, healthy adults, the infection can be devastating in pregnant women or people infected with HIV. It has been estimated that some 3,300 congenitally infected children are born in the United States each year, for direct costs of some $430 million. In Europe and North America, 10 to 30 percent of people with AIDS have died of brain infections with *Toxoplasma*. This occurrence has, in some misguided medical quarters, raised an unwarranted fear of proximity to cats; there is no evidence that owning a cat puts one at risk.

The scientific evidence suggests that most people get toxoplasmosis from eating undercooked meat, especially pork or lamb. The pigs and sheep get it from their feed, which is contaminated by cats on the farms, who use the feed bins as giant litter boxes. The cats probably pick the parasite up from wild mice. The biggest reported outbreak ever (several thousand people) was in Victoria, British Columbia; that was waterborne. The water was infected by either mountain lions or feral cats in the watershed.

One might think, based on ecological or fecal grounds, that parasitic diseases such as trichinosis or toxoplasmosis would be geographically restricted. How far can a carnivore go, after all, to complete a parasitic life cycle? As your inquiring minds will have noticed, however, parasites, and not just bacteria and viruses, have found ways to take advantage of new global travel packages that our species offers them. One in particular opens a larger window into how we might begin to think differently about our food system.

In the spring of 1996, and again in the spring of 1997, government health authorities in Canada and the United States received reports of outbreaks of gastrointestinal disease involving a total of more than two thousand people in various cities throughout the continent. Clinical signs included long-term (one to three weeks) diarrhea, loss of appetite, abdominal pain, nausea, vomiting, fever, and, not surprisingly, given the other symptoms, fatigue and weight loss.

The cause of this abdominal discomfort appeared to be a relatively unknown single-celled parasite, *Cyclospora cayetensis*. The first human cases had been reported in 1979, and most scientists knew little about it. About a week after ingesting a cyclospora oocyst, the victim usually comes down with watery diarrhea and frequent, sometimes explosive stools. An infected person may be sick for a month if left untreated, shedding oocysts in his or her feces. These oocysts take a couple of days to weeks to become infectious for other people, so the infection spreads through environmental contamination rather than directly person to person. Related species of *Cyclospora* have been found in rodents and reptiles; the same species has been cultured from a duck in Peru and from a group of Mexican chickens. The disease in people can be treated with sulfa drugs.

Initial reports suggested that the vehicle for the parasite was strawberries from California. In July 1996, a meeting was held at the Centers for Disease Control and Prevention in the United States, attended by representatives of various levels of government, as well as universities, from Canada and the United States. Summaries of disease investigations after that meeting identified Guatemalan raspberries as the primary food vehicle in most outbreaks, along with, in a few outbreaks, mesclun (a mixture of various types of baby lettuce). Later reports do not mention strawberries. Not surprisingly, Guatemalan farmers and their representatives, who were not at the meeting, accused U.S. scientists of biased judgments intended to protect California strawberry growers. In 1998, the Food and Drug Administration did not allow Guatemalan raspberries into the United States; Canada did. That year Canada, but not the United States, had outbreaks of *Cyclospora* infection. Since then, both blackberries and snow peas from Guatemala have been implicated.

Although the medical description of disease behavior had some immediate diagnostic use, and the foods and their sources gave public health officials some options for prevention, the situation has proved to be more complicated and systemic than a simple case of feces in the food supply might suggest.

The Institute of Medicine (IOM) in the United States has proposed that the causes of the emergence of new infectious diseases such as cyclosporiasis include changes in human demographics and behavior; technology, industry, and commerce; international travel; economic development and land use; the breakdown of public health measures; and microbial adaptation. Using this list of causes, we might come up with a list of possible reasons that this disease emerged as a problem.

1. Human demographics and behavior have changed dramatically in the last few decades in Latin America. As population densities in the countryside increase, young people in particular have migrated from the countryside to city slums, looking for employment. International trade agreements, coupled with programs to promote nontraditional export crops such as snow peas, broccoli, and raspberries, provide one avenue for generating foreign exchange that could be used to finance economic development and, perhaps, to create employment. At the same time, changing diets in the United States and Canada provide opportunities for marketing some of those export crops.

2. Consolidation and mass distribution in agribusiness is a natural consequence of economic market forces. Improved technology enables these businesses to ship fragile fruits such as raspberries over long distances to take advantage of off-season markets.

3. Not only are people traveling to more places, but also, as a result of multinational trade agreements, more food is traveling.

4. Land use practices in many poor tropical countries reflect a mix of traditional farmers, large, wealthy land holders, and many smaller, impoverished farmers. Given the economic gains to be had from economies of scale, it is not surprising that these conventional land ownership patterns have resisted land reform programs and, indeed, have been reinforced. The case of cyclosporiasis and raspberries indicates that the implications of these land ownership patterns are relevant not only to local politics but also to public health issues far removed from the farms.

5. Much of the public health infrastructure that was built up in the industrialized world after World War II is now aging, but less money is being put into the system to rejuvenate it. As a result, food surveillance and inspection in receiving countries

as well as in the countries of origin are not keeping pace with the rise in food trade.

6. Bacteria, viruses, and parasites can adapt to new ecological conditions as quickly as we can create them and more quickly than we can devise ways to control them. The raspberry export schemes provided an ecological opportunity for dissemination.

But the situation is even more complicated than this list of causes might suggest. In North America, an aging postwar generation concerned about its health is eating more fruits and vegetables, which are transported long distances from economically disadvantaged southern countries. North American consumers, abetted by big-box supermarkets, are accustomed to low prices in grocery stores, and so economies of scale, corporate concentration of ownership, and economic disparities in countries such as Guatemala are reinforced. Thus, North American diets have placed contradictory pressures on the world agrifood system; most of these pressures spring from the desire to improve personal health and save money, at the unintended expense of the global public good. The facts are not controversial, nor are the systemic effects on disease emergence part of some conspiracy. Agrifood companies are doing what they are there for, making money for shareholders, regardless of the cost. What is, or should be, a source of considerable controversy is the blithe obliviousness of North American food consumers to the effects of their daily dietary choices, and the lack of political will to even talk about what trade-offs we are making when we eat and what it might mean to behave as decent global citizens.

In March 1999, I was bouncing along in an old yellow Guatemalan Blue Bird school bus repainted in brilliant reds and blues and yellows, squeezed into a seat intended for two, now accommodating a short, wizened man in a cowboy hat and bright red trousers, two Mayan women with babies peering over their shoulders from tightly patterned, intricately woven cotton slings, and me, baskets and bags piled on our laps. I watch the landscape of medieval-looking Spanish towns, volcanoes, and huge Pepsi-Cola signs slip by. Seeing the backbreakingly steep fields clawing their way up the mountainsides into the forests, I found it hard to imagine that Guatemala exported over US$300 million worth of fresh fruits and vegetables, primarily to North America, in 1996. And this on top of nearly a billion dollars in traditional crops such as coffee, sugar, tobacco, and bananas.

In Guatemala, over half the children are malnourished, infectious diseases are rampant, Vitamin A and iodine and iron deficiencies are widespread, and the infant mortality rate is six times that of Cuba and almost nine times that of Canada. Why would this country ship huge amounts of food to North America? How do we put together the insights of the Institute of Medicine with the complexity of real-world interactions?

In the early 1980s, the Reagan administration in the United States was in the midst of a war on both military and political fronts to defend American interests in the region. On the military front, the United States supported the military leaders of Guatemala in such a way that they were able to carry out Kosovo-style ethnic cleansing, massacring men, women, and children in some 450 mostly indigenous Maya villages. At the same time, with help from the U.S. Agency for International Development and the Caribbean Basin Initiative, Guatemalan farmers were lured toward a bright future, which the distinctive American version of free enterprise would create for them. Switching from corn and beans, which were good only for local markets and provided no occasion to generate foreign exchange, Guatemalan farmers were persuaded to grow raspberries for export in the anticipation of higher incomes. Some of them may have wondered (though this is pure speculation on my part) if their newfound raspberry wealth might help them beat the annual spring epidemic of stomach problems in their children.

After all, more money can buy better nutrition, and better nutrition means stronger immune systems to fight off disease.

The Guatemalan initiative was well timed to take advantage of some radical changes in the North American diet, the response of an aging, health-conscious baby boomer generation to epidemiological studies demonstrating the health benefits of eating more fresh fruits and vegetables. These dietary changes were already being inserted into a postwar agrifood system whose primary goal was to provide large amounts of food at low cost. This combination opened opportunities for a variety of specialty fruits and vegetables that could be grown in the tropics but were only seasonally available in North America. The Guatemalan entry into the North American raspberry market also coincided with a political atmosphere of deregulation and disinvestment in public health infrastructure, which, among other things, minimized food inspection. None of these interacting elements provided an incentive to provide training, good pay, and good hygiene facilities for field workers in Guatemala.

Between 1992 and 1996, Guatemalans increased their annual raspberry exports to the United States from 4,000 to 700,000 pounds. Although this export boom did not eradicate the Guatemalans' own disease problems, it did help them share their burden with several thousand Americans and Canadians. Some public health officials noticed that the people affected appeared to be mostly relatively wealthy people at business luncheons and weddings—that is, those who could afford to serve raspberries out of season. There is some irony in the fact that many of these people are from the socioeconomic class that most strongly supported the market-based economic agenda that resulted in the epidemic.

To say that any one of these is the cause of the cyclosporiasis emergence is to miss the point. The various elements tend to organize themselves into particular patterns of feedback loops, over a range of temporal and spatial scales. These patterns represent more or less self-organizing systems; that is, the elements—importers, raspberry growers, consumers, parasites—interact in such a way that the loops begin to close in on themselves and reinforce each other. Although conscious human decisions play important roles in these systems, this consciousness is usually focused on immediate considerations and does not recognize or address links to overall system effects. Disease patterns such as those involved in the emergence of cyclosporiasis are embedded in these self-organizing systems.

Once we recognize these systemic feedback loops, what can we do about them? How can we manage these kinds of food-borne diseases with a sense of international goodwill, solidarity, and good science? I will come back to these questions in the last two chapters of the book.

8

ZOMBIES
FROM
THE
DEEP

SEAFOOD TOXINS

AFTER INVESTIGATING the nature and origins of zombie stories in Haiti, ethnobot-
anist Wade Davis suggested that at least
one ingredient in creating zombism was something called tetrodotoxin. This toxin affects the sodium channels in nerves that
stimulate certain muscles in the body—the voluntary ones,
such as those in your eyelids or the ones you use for breathing.
The heart keeps beating and your eyelids remain fixed as you
are put into a coffin and lowered into the ground. Not surprisingly, when a kind vodun priest digs you up the next night, you
may be in a state of shock. You might even do whatever he tells
you to. You certainly won't be a troublemaker in the community
anymore.

One might forgive religious leaders for drawing on their knowledge of natural toxins to keep the flock in line, but the culinary tales about tetrodotoxin are both more mundane and stranger than vodun religion.

In April 1996, a twenty-three-year-old chef in California ate a small piece of fugu. About fifteen minutes later, his mouth and lips tingled. Then he felt dizzy and tired. Then his throat constricted, he had trouble speaking, he started shaking, and he threw up. Finally, his legs gave out and he collapsed. He was one of three chefs who sampled this Japanese delicacy, which had been smuggled into the United States. Thanks to good emergency medical treatment, all three men survived.

The Japanese have developed a taste for various kinds of puffer fish that contain high concentrations of tetrodotoxin. The toxin is produced by member of the *Vibrio* bacterial family and is found in high concentrations in puffer fish, porcupine fish, and fugu, as well as blue-ringed octopi, California newts, and eastern salamanders. Why the chefs didn't just eat an American salamander is beyond me; it would seem to offer a similar sense of extreme culinary adventure.

Like many fish toxins, tetrodotoxin accumulates in the reproductive organs and intestines of the fish; if cleaned properly, the flesh is safe. The Japanese have a system of certified puffer fish cleaners and, very occasionally, are allowed to export to Japanese restaurants in the United States under special permits. China, Japan, the Philippines, Taiwan, and Mexico all allow export of the fish.

Since a small portion prepared by a professional might cost US$400, some frugal gourmands might avail themselves of an unofficial (street?) cleaner. He may even be as good as an official one. If you have bad luck in this game of culinary roulette, however, your fingers and toes tingle, you bleed internally, your skin peels off, your muscles twitch, your eyes remain fixed, and eventually you are paralyzed. Sixty percent of the people who eat the toxin in its concentrated form die. About fifty people a year die from eating the fish in Japan.

A Japanese gourmand might argue that the food is worth both a professional cleaner and the $400 and that the probability of dying after eating puffer fish is probably less than that of dying in a motorbike accident on your way to the local convenience store. If one is going to die for food, it might be said, one must just as well die with valor.

The other option for the intrepid North American eater is to catch the fish yourself. In 2002 about ten people in Florida, New Jersey, and Virginia fell ill with tetrodotoxin poisoning after eating fish caught near Titusville, Florida. Although toxic puffer fish were known to swim off the Baja peninsula on the Pacific coast of North America, these were the first cases of toxic puffer fish in the Atlantic. Fortunately, the concentrations of toxin were not as great as those found in the South Pacific waters, and all of the adventurous eaters survived.

Fugu poisoning is not the only danger lurking in marine waters.

Not too many years ago, many of us thought water was safe, and seafood was hailed as the centerpiece of many health food diets. Today we know that seafood is no safer than any other type of food. In fact, some medical researchers have called for bans on the serving of aquatic foods such as raw shellfish, which are particularly dangerous. The ancient Egyptians and Israelites could have warned us: ". . . and all the water that was in the Nile turned to blood. And the fish in the Nile died; and the Nile became foul, so that the Egyptians could not drink from the Nile . . ."

The Italian novelist Primo Levi might also have written about shellfish as a kind of fruit from the Tree of Knowledge. The plague of the water-turned-to-blood visited upon the ancient Egyptians might have been what we call today a red tide, a bloom of tiny plantlike animals called dinoflagellates. If so, then at least some of the apparently arbitrary rules laid out in Mosaic law about clean and unclean food may be seen as both food safety regulations and an act of cultural identity.

Dinoflagellate blooms may be accompanied by spectacular displays of nighttime luminescence. The Pacific coast Indians in North America didn't know about the chemistry of saxitoxins, which are related to tetrodotoxins but occur in shellfish. They did know, however, that algal blooms were a warning from nature not to eat the shellfish, which became toxic at such times. This warning system is not perfect, but it's not bad. Not all "red tides" are red. They may be violet, orange, blue, green, or invisible, and not all are toxic.

On June 15, 1793, four members of Captain George Vancouver's ship's crew went hunting for mussels on the rocky beach along the west coast of what is now British Columbia. Had they been on better speaking terms with the local inhabitants, they might have learned some tricks for checking the safety of these tasty bivalves. They might even have been warned by the locals to avoid certain beaches at certain times. But these white men, knowing what was good, as white men always do, had no need to ask help of anyone and suffered the consequences: paralytic shellfish poisoning. One of them, John Carter, died in respiratory distress five hours after eating the mussels. The other three survived. This episode shows once again that not asking questions (1) is a male thing and (2) may have bad consequences. Of course, it only proves this if you believe that one carefully selected case is sufficient evidence to hang a theory on.

Almost two hundred years later, in the same general area, a husband and wife spent a pleasant few hours shucking clams on Porter's Beach, British Columbia. They tossed the black siphon tips to their cats, and the man nibbled on one of the raw clams. A couple of hours later, he felt his lips and tongue becoming numb, and he watched in horror as both cats became sick and one died. The man was lucky; he had given the most toxic part to the cats, and he scraped by with a mere warning.

Although Paralytic Shellfish Poisoning (PSP) occurs sporadically, it served, until a few years ago, as the main rationale behind testing shellfish by public health laboratories in North America. These laboratories target high-risk areas for periodic testing of shellfish for the PSP toxins. If a mouse into which an extract of the shellfish is injected dies within fifteen minutes, then it is probably not good for people. Two to three weeks after a bloom, the shellfish are usually safe, except for certain types, such as butter clams, which may hoard the saxitoxin for up to two years. The toxin is not destroyed by cooking.

The fifteen-minute mouse test was the standard for the industry until 1987. Late that year, and well into the next, a series of patients entered hospitals in Montreal with nausea, vomiting, diarrhea, headaches, and, in some cases, disorientation, slurred speech, memory loss, seizures, and coma. The disease was linked epidemiologically to the consumption of Prince Edward Island's famous blue mussels. Political and public panic, with subsequent closure of the East Coast shellfish industry and economic panic, was accompanied by very intense laboratory and field investigations. Scientists concluded that the human disease was due to a chemical called domoic acid. This acid fools our bodies into believing that it is a substance that our bodies need and want, but once in the door, instead of being the friendly grandmother, glutamic acid, it behaves like a neurological wolf. Like all reputable toxins, this one has practical uses as well. Domoic-acid-like substances extracted from seaweed by Chinese and Japanese herbalists are sold in the Far East as antiworm medication for children.

Unfortunately for the East Coast shellfish growers, the fifteen-minute mouse test does not work on domoic acid. The mice behaved abnormally, and they did die, but not until an hour after being injected, a fact that was allegedly discovered (as many scientific facts are) by accident, accompanied by close observation and reflection. In fact, the chemical does not appear to be as toxic in the laboratory as it should be to wreak the havoc it is purported to. As a result, scientists question whether it really is the culprit. Since those initial outbreaks in Prince Edward Island, scientists have developed better tests (thus better protecting public health), but have also discovered that domoic acid problems are not confined to Canada's east coast, nor are their effects just related to human health. Domoic acid levels associated with algal blooms have been increasing in size and frequency off the coast of California since the early 1990s. These blooms have sickened and killed thousands of birds, and marine mammals such as whales and sea lions. Surviving sea lions, like the human survivors, may have permanent brain damage. The causes of these increases in domoic acid are likely a systemic mix of increasing pollution (fertilizer runoff, paint washed off boats) and global warming.

DOMOIC ACID is not the only—and probably not the most important—marine toxin resulting from our aggressive messing with natural systems. On the evening of March 27, 1987, sixty Canadian tourists were celebrating cross-cultural warmth at a Cuban hotel. As a last meal before returning to northern jobs and overcast skies, the sun followers partook of a Caribbean fish casserole. Two to six hours later, in flight back to Montreal, thirty-eight of these culinary migrants came down with nausea, vomiting, and/or abdominal pain with, according to the *Canadian Diseases Weekly Report* (an official publication of Health Canada), "understandable stress on the aeroplane's sanitary facilities." Within eight to forty-eight hours after eating the fish, more than fifty of the tourists began suffering neurological symptoms, including tingling sensations around the mouth, numbness, severe itching, burning sensations on the hands and feet and in the mouth, headaches, insomnia, muscle pains, and extreme weakness. The strangest signs for this disease include a feeling that one's teeth are loose and the reversal of hot and cold, so that a warm shower feels freezing and ice cream tastes burningly hot. For most, the gastrointestinal symptoms cleared up in a few days; the neurological problems persisted for weeks.

Ciguatera fish poisoning, which is what the Canadian tourists in Cuba had, is also related to accumulations of toxins in microscopic marine creatures. Although the toxins have been found in over four hundred species of fish, human intoxications are most often related to the consumption of reef fish at the top of the food chain, mostly grouper, barracuda, red snapper, amberjack, and kingfish, but also moray eels.

Ciguatoxin—or rather, ciguatoxins, since there is a whole family of them—is 22,000 times as toxic (to mice, and presumably to people) as cyanide. Its effects are therefore felt at very tiny doses, meaning that the "toxic" fish only contain minute amounts of the poisons. Researchers have tried for years to characterize the toxins; Japanese researchers used four and a half tons of moray eels to extract about one one-hundredth of an ounce of one of the ciguatoxins, a figure that tells you something about animal sacrifice to the gods of personal health. Since then, the Japanese researchers have found ways to synthesize a couple of the other toxins in the laboratory (a feat that, presumably, requires a smaller amount of lab space and fewer complaints from colleagues down the hall about the smell). The reason that scientists want to determine the molecular structure of these toxins is so that they can create tests to detect toxins in the fish before people eat them, as well as tests for making a diagnosis in people, which now relies on a mixture of eating history and odd clinical signs.

Anyone with culinary ties to the latitudes between 35° north and 35° south may succumb to this disease. Ciguatera poisoning was first described by Europeans in the Caribbean and South

Pacific in the sixteenth century, but people knew about it long before that. In the Caribbean, the cause of the illness was first ascribed to a shrub, *el manzanillo*, that grows on riverbanks. The name probably comes from a univalve mollusc that the Cubans call *cigua*, which lives around coral reefs; people who got sick after eating *cigua* were called *ciguatos*, and the term was later applied to anyone who got sick after eating seafood. From such ambiguous beginnings, and still shrouded in many scientific uncertainties, ciguatera fish poisoning has risen in importance to become the most commonly reported marine intoxication in the world. In the 1990s, there were over a thousand cases in Hong Kong alone. While people who live next to seas with coral reefs can easily catch their own poisons, those who live farther away need to make some effort. Canadians tend to acquire the disease by importing fish from their favorite reefs in the Caribbean, the Indian Ocean, and the South Pacific. Although it is illegal to sell barracuda for food in Florida, it's legal to sell it out of state—to Canada, for instance, or California. What was it P.T. Barnum said about suckers?

Although the primary means of getting the intoxication is through food, there are reports that ciguatera poisoning has been transmitted through heterosexual contact, both male to female and female to male. The men, on top of all their other symptoms, developed penile pain; the women got pelvic and abdominal pain. Ciguatera is the only foodborne infection for which I have been able to find evidence of transmission through the orifices used in heterosexual genital-to-genital contact. Once you begin to play with other orifices, all bets are off. Just about anything that goes through the digestive tract can be— and has been—transmitted.

People who have experienced ciguatera toxicity once often get it worse the next time. Strangely, this secondary reaction can be triggered by almost any seafood, as well as by nuts and alcohol. Wild partying, it turns out, cannot be used to make the bad feelings go away.

That ciguatoxins cause disease is clear, but what causes ciguatoxins to develop? Here the picture gets considerably more complex. The dinoflagellates that contain the ciguatoxins are eaten by small fish, which accumulate the toxins in their bodies (a process called bioaccumulation) over a lifetime of eating. These small fish are eaten by larger fish, which accumulate the toxin already accumulated by the smaller fish from the dinoflagellates. Thus, at each stage of the food pyramid, the poison is further concentrated in a process called biomagnification. The dinoflagellates involved in this process apparently have a fondness for living among macroalgae (the big leafy ones), which is what grows when coral reefs are damaged. These processes of bioaccumuation and biomagnification explain why many toxins (such as organochlorine pesticides and radionuclides) go from low concentrations in the general environment to high concentrations in particular foods.

Coral reefs are damaged by warming of ocean temperatures (as a result of global warming from burning all those fossil fuels), nutrient runoff from coastal areas (sewage from cities, industrial waste, agricultural runoff), direct damage from tourists scrunching around to see what's under their floppy feet, nuclear tests in the South Pacific designed to make the world safe for the reef scrunchers, and overfishing for both food for hungry people and ornamental fish for the reef scrunchers so that when they get home they can feel nostalgic for what once was. Disease, after all, is simply another name for natural consequences. Medicine is the art of contextualizing it.

In the 1990s, when the Soviet Union collapsed and Cuba was set adrift, the Cubans went into what was called the "special period." People were starving and ate whatever they could get their hands on, including some of the larger reef fish. Karen

Morrison, a member of our research team and a graduate student who worked with me, investigated how the sportfishers, public health authorities, and ecological researchers dealt with this situation and the possibility of intoxication.

Given that the Cubans had no money and no fancy backup from North America, they did amazingly well. Many of the physicians were able to put together diagnoses based on clinical signs and the eating history of patients. The professional fishers were pretty good at figuring things out and wouldn't put friends or family at risk. Since there are no good laboratory tests for ciguatera toxins, they tried things like tasting a little or feeding a piece to a cat and watching what happened. Sometimes—like the Floridians selling toxic fish to Montreal restaurants—illegal fishers would sneak out onto the water in small craft, snag a few big fish, and then sell them in pieces on the street in cities like Havana. In our workshops there, we came across some amazing instances in which schoolchildren mobilized to educate their communities about conservation and health issues. Real progress wasn't made in controlling the human disease, however, until the economy began picking up in the new millennium.

Throughout the world, dealing effectively with ciguatera poisoning has been hampered by an uncertain understanding of its basic ecology, the lack of good diagnostic tests, and the multilayered, multifaceted causal web within which it has emerged. Its causes are individual, national, and global; they are economic, political, climatic, ecological, and dietary. Ciguatera poisoning really doesn't fit into our neat categories of "this" causes "that" and therefore, quite simply, "this" must be stopped.

If infection with *Salmonella* is part of a global pandemic with a long reach into the past, then intoxication with ciguatera, with its connections to global warming, imports, sex, reefs, and uncertain laboratory results, is the wave of the future. There are two lessons here. One is that diseases such as ciguatera can only be dealt with in the long run if ecologists, public health investigators, and fishers work together. The other is that if people cannot harvest fish for food or money, they need alternatives.

A 1986 editorial in the *New England Journal of Medicine* asked: "Consumption of raw shellfish—is the risk now unacceptable?" This apparently rhetorical question was in response to reports that over a thousand people had gotten sick from eating shellfish in New York State over an eight-month period. If there are toxins in the water—whether they be mercury, ciguatera, or domoic acid—filter-feeding shellfish (clams, oysters, scallops, and cockles) will accumulate them. They will also collect any available bacteria, such as the vibrios that cause cholera, or whatever viruses have been pooped out by our cities into the pollution dilution tank.

In theory, we have in place a system that protects consumers. Shellfish from certain areas are either all of the time (because of bacterial or chemical pollution) or some of the time (because of dinoflagellate poisons) classified as unsafe for human consumption. In some cases, a process called depuration is used. Depuration is a kind of detox program for intoxicated shellfish. Shellfish that might be marginally safe are placed in tanks of water that is either naturally clean or have been cleaned with ozone or ultraviolet light. The shellfish are left there to cleanse themselves for two or three days. A tag showing the source of the shellfish is supposed to follow them to retailers and restaurants. Depuration is not always effective, however, and, as in the case of the domoic acid, nature may confound us with new toxins. The most serious problems, however, invariably come back to the willingness of pure-blooded capitalists to take risks with other people's lives. Tags get lost or switched around.

In an age of multinational capitalism, government regulation is essential to the well-being of world society. Perhaps nowhere does the pollution of the commons affect us as much as in marine systems. Even if we manage the fragile art of obtaining safe foods from water, we cannot let down our guard. In 1985, Canadian tuna that had been declared unfit for human consumption was sold to a company in the United States for cat food; several transactions and label changes later, in 1992, the cans were crossing the border back into Canada as human food. Regulatory vigilance is always necessary and appropriate. At the same time, we could regulate ourselves to death. Somewhere out there is a balance between vigilance against fraud and acceptance of fate, between laws of the sea and respect for the sea, between global community and local control. If we do not attain that balance, it should not be said that it was for want of trying.

WHEN SHE

—

MOVES IN

9

ARE WE SAFE YET?

TRANSFORMING DANGER

INTO RISK

PEOPLE USED to talk about danger. Some time in the 1980s and 1990s, scientists began to talk about the public's "perceived" risk of dangers of chemical residues in food. This was followed by an explosion of scientific and governmental literature trying to define and measure "real" risks and to use those as a basis for national and international regulation of trade in food. Danger is what people feel. Risk is what technocrats manage. Perceived risks, so the theory went, are what people have when they don't understand what is "real." Having set out the parameters of the discussions, scientists were left with one problem: what, exactly, was real?

Foodborne-disease-reporting systems are designed to pick up only acute, and not chronic, chemical intoxications. Acute chemical intoxications, like acute disease caused by bacterial toxins, almost always occur within minutes to hours of ingestion of the contaminated or toxic food. Although the specific clinical signs vary from one toxin to another, some generalizations are possible. When the toxins hit the stomach, they usually cause nausea and vomiting, together with generalized or nervous-system-related signs. For these acute intoxications, the real and the perceived tend to pretty much coincide, the people afflicted complain, and the surveillance systems have little trouble identifying the problem.

On July 10, 1981, a group of students at a small college in San Bernardino, California, sat down to brunch. It was the usual student fare, the kind of low-cost concoction you would try out at second weaning, like zucchini cake. About an hour after brunch, some of the students were feeling dizzy, anxious, confused, and drowsy; a few felt their hearts race and their limbs tingle and then, in midsentence, forgot exactly what wonderful thing they were expounding on to this incredibly beautiful person beside them. Later, the preparer of the zucchini cake confessed to health officials that he may have inadvertently added marijuana to the recipe.

In September 1983, a man was admitted to hospital in Edmonton, Alberta, with vomiting, dry mouth, dizziness, double vision, and delirium. His condition, and that of a Toronto woman the same year but half a country away, was traced to a little too much of a good thing: an herbal tea containing the natural drug atropine.

On October 8, 1983, Mrs. Gabriella Toews (a fictional name) decided to fix hamburgers for supper. In order to spruce up this somewhat ordinary American meal, she reached up, pulled down a bottle of seasoning from the shelf, and sprinkled some over the meat. She then realized that the seasoning she had used was in fact seeds of angels' trumpets (*Datura suaveolens*) that she had been drying above the stove. Annoyed and frugal to the last, she carefully picked out the seeds and went on with getting supper ready. Less than an hour after eating his hamburger, and just as he was settling into his tea and the newspaper, George Toews thought the page before him was swimming with strange shapes. He felt his mouth go dry and then, clutching his stomach, ran for the toilet. He passed out. Gabriella's heart was racing as she struggled to make out the telephone number for the ambulance. By the time it arrived, she too was unconscious.

On February 12, 1987, several people in British Columbia got sick from drinking "blue pop" from a vending machine. A malfunction of the machine had caused carbonated water to flow through copper piping and leached copper out of the pipes. Acute cases of metal toxicity can occur when acid foods (fruit juices, tomato juice, carbonated beverages) dissolve the metal containers in which they are being kept. Salts of metals can be corrosive and so they irritate the lining of your stomach and result in vomiting.

In North America, these are typical of the kinds of incidents—along with the story of the Quebec woman who slipped strychnine into her husband's vitamin pills to put him out of her misery—which comprise many of the reported incidents of chemical poisoning in the government reports on foodborne illness.

Occasionally, foodborne reporting systems pick up acute intoxications on a larger scale. Sometimes they are absurd and economically important but not real health issues. The case of the Austrian wine makers who added antifreeze to their wine to sweeten it comes to mind. Antifreeze is indeed sweet, which is why animals love it, and it can destroy your kidneys, which is why animals need to be kept away from it, but both the form and the doses of the antifreeze in the wine were not of major public health importance. One public health official estimated you would need to drink twenty-eight bottles a day for two weeks to get sick. But one might ask, if you did that, would you even notice that you were sick?

Other reported instances are more serious. In the 1980s, in the United States, people, mostly women, began showing up at doctors' offices with severe muscle pain. The laboratory tests showed that one type of white blood cell, the eosinophils, appeared in their blood in high numbers. Michael Osterholme and his team of epidemiologists at the Minnesota Department of Health tracked the cause of eosinophilia-myalgia syndrome, as it came to be called. The trail led to a Japanese factory, where a batch of an amino acid called L-tryptophan, sold in health food stores to be used for such ailments as insomnia and depression, had been made. More than a thousand people got sick, and a couple of dozen of them died. The fact that the supplement was produced by genetically modified organisms (GMOs) did not do much to spiffy up the international image of these organisms.

And then there was the infamous Spanish toxic oil syndrome. On May 1, 1981, an eight-year-old boy in Madrid died of what looked like pneumonia. In the weeks that followed, thousands of patients began to show up in Spanish hospitals with coughing, chest pain, headaches, and fever. Within a year, more than twenty thousand people had fallen ill with this strange disease, and more than three hundred victims had died.

The outbreak generated many investigations and several major reports published by the World Health Organization. The Spanish government, protecting its olive oil industry, had a policy requiring that imported rapeseed (now called canola) oils be treated with aniline, an organic substance used in manufacturing dyes and polyurethane, so that they would be unusable for human consumption. Unrepentant capitalists (this was, after all, the Reagan-Thatcher era in world economics) then took some of this oil and treated it to make it—so they thought—fit for people. They then mixed this "detoxified" oil with olive oil and sold it as pure olive oil at bargain prices to poor consumers. Like well-trained consumers everywhere, the customers thought that getting something cheaper was always a good thing. I recall buying "pure corn oil" in Indonesia during the same time period; it turned solid when I put it into the refrigerator (which corn oil would not do).

Sporadic (nonoutbreak), acute intoxications are so uncommon that many countries don't even include them in their published reports of foodborne diseases. It is no wonder, then, that some food safety experts view chemical residue problems as a minor concern. The low numbers and sporadic occurrence of acute chemical intoxications, however, do not reflect the real effects. For the most part, scientists are concerned about *chronic* exposure to substances such as heavy metals, dioxins, and antibiotics. Furthermore, the outcomes that interest consumers—cancers, reproductive problems—have complex causes. Systems that monitor foodborne diseases are not designed to detect these outcomes, however, so that any statement about the relative risks of chemicals versus infectious agents based on the surveillance system is really a load of manure.

The world is made of chemicals, as are you and I. The American Chemical Society had registered more than four million chemicals by the end of the 1970s and was adding about six thousand a week to the list. People have had intimate relationships with chemicals, sometimes with adverse consequences, for as long as we have been around. Modern industry and agriculture, however, have accelerated the rate at which chemicals are concentrated and redistributed around the world. Sulfur from Chile and potash from Saskatchewan go to American farmlands, Siberian uranium goes to Europe, and so on. This redistribution, combined with the introduction of five hundred to seven hundred new manufactured compounds every year over the past few decades, has disturbed this evolutionary equilibrium, often dramatically. No wonder people are concerned about chemical pollution and chemical-producing industries. Although people can be exposed to chemicals by various means, food is the dominant route of exposure for a large class of organic chemicals, many of which, such as PCB and DDT, have been used in agricultural and industrial activities.

Technically, consideration of chemicals in food could include everything from biological toxins active naturally in some foods (mushroom poisonings, paralytic shellfish toxins) to agricultural and industrial chemicals that find their way into the food chain. One could add a discussion on food additives that have inadvertently been added at the wrong "dose," overdoses of some herbal teas, or additives that have intentionally been used, such as strychnine added to vitamin pills.

Before we dive into the scientific idea of risk, it is useful to separate the toxins produced by nonhuman life forms, sometimes called "natural" toxins, from "chemicals," toxins manufactured by people. These terms imply that humans are not natural, however, which, biologically speaking, is a nonstarter. Everything is natural, that is, of nature. However, toxins produced by bacteria (botulism) or dinoflagellates (ciguatera), or fungi (which are covered in chapter 12) tell us different things about the nature of food safety than toxins such as pesticides (discussed in chapter 10) produced by people for specific purposes.

Heavy metals (covered in more detail in chapter 11) are a special case. Humans don't create them, but we do concentrate and distribute them in ways that severely challenge both ecosystems and human health. Although they are a major global concern (think of lead in water or canned food, or mercury in fish), one could write several tomes to cover them all, and defined outbreaks are rare. The postwar Japanese have suffered through major self-inflicted experiments with mercury poisoning (dancing cat disease) at Minamata and cadmium toxicity (also called *itai-itai*, or ouch-ouch, disease because of the sore and brittle bones it causes.) Despite convincing evidence from Japan, people have sometimes tried to replicate the experiment elsewhere (mercury at Grassy Narrows in Canada), as if some perverse scientist were asking the question: yes, it's bad in Japanese people, but does that mean it's bad in Canadians?

Among the manufactured chemicals, pesticides have raised the greatest concerns and have had the most influence on how scientific risk came to be defined. And among the pesticides, the organochlorines (with names such as DDT, aldrin, dieldrin, and chlordane) have raised the loudest alarm bells. As I explained when talking about ciguatera toxicity, the problem with these substances is that they bioaccumulate and biomagnify—that is, they accumulate in the fat of animals that are continuously exposed to them, and then, as the big animals eat the little ones, their concentrations are increased up the food chain.

In one experiment, done when such experiments were still considered acceptable, a form of DDT was applied to a lake at 0.02 ppm (parts per million). Within a year, the concentration in plankton was at 10 ppm, little fish at 900 ppm, and large fish and fish-eating birds at 2,000 ppm. Also, because they accumulate in fat, these substances end up in human breast milk. Although regulations in North America have put strict controls on the use of these substances, they are still entering the food chain on a global scale; what the long-term effects on people will be is unknown. Some, like DDT, are apparently safe for people. The effects on other members of the ecosystem, especially birds, we already know to be devastating.

In some cases, toxic chemicals are deliberately, and illegally, added to food; for example, antifreeze (ethylene glycol) may be added to wine as a sweetener. Intentional food additives may be added in the wrong amounts or may have chronic effects even at the "right" amounts. Some of these, such as nitrites or niacin, are incorporated at processing; others, such as MSG, are usually added during the preparation of the food. I'll talk about food additives in a later chapter, but right now, I want to get back to how scientists assess these sorts of chemicals in general.

Given all this stuff out there, it would be surprising if people did not have a sense of danger. And if the normal foodborne-disease–reporting system does not tell us much, how can we study this issue, or talk about it intelligently? How does one begin to transform the vague sense of danger from all the stuff we are making, and to which our bodies have evolved no adaptations, into something scientific, measurable, and manageable? Faced with this question, scientists created something called risk analysis.

Risk analysis has three parts: risk assessment, risk communication, and risk management. It sounds relatively straightforward and abstract and scientific. Bear with me. It gets both messy and interesting.

Risk assessment is a way of summarizing what scientists know, or think they know, about the risks various chemicals pose to us. Risk assessment is also a way of bringing together value judgments and scientific data to enable people to make decisions. The results of risk assessment should not, under any circumstances, be confused with "hard facts," although spokespeople for both chemical industries and consumer advocacy groups may present them as such.

The risk assessment process includes four steps. The first step is called hazard identification. Is the substance we are considering a hazard, that is, can it cause biological damage to people? The second step was originally called dose-response assessment and called upon scientists to determine if the negative effect of the substance was related to the dose consumed. Now this step is referred to as hazard characterization. An assessment of the relationship between dose and response is still core to this step; however, while the originators of risk assessment saw this as being a quantitative measurement, more qualitative judgments about the nature of this relationship are now allowed. At the third step, exposure assessment, scientists look at how much of the hazardous substance people are actually getting into their systems. For the final step, risk characterization, they take all the information and put it together into a report they can present to policymakers. Is this substance in our food supply something we should be concerned about?

Risk assessment is the most scientifically based of the three parts of risk analysis. Although risk assessment separates the hazard part from the dose, the words of the sixteenth-century Swiss physician Paracelsus are appropriate: "What is it that is not a poison? All things are poison and nothing is without poison. It is the dose only that makes a thing not a poison." Thus, for instance, veterinarians give cows a stomach stimulant that contains the parent compound for strychnine, and enough children have overdosed on aspirin for us to know that our best wonder cures can kill us. Some industrial spokespeople like to use this argument when discussing the toxicity of potatoes and peanut butter, implying that manufactured chemicals are, in comparison, relatively harmless. That argument, which I shall return to later, misses the point.

There are, nevertheless, some very real problems in assessing chemical hazards in foods. In the first place, what kinds of effects are scientists looking for? The most commonly measured effect is cancer, but one might just as well look for reproductive, neurobehavioral, and immunological changes. In the case of chemical residues, one adds an extra twist. The victim dies a decade or two later. Now find the culprit. What were you eating ten years ago? What was in that food? Have you done anything since then that might have compromised your body? Would you admit it if you had?

Second, investigators need to have some preconceived idea about how common a problem is before they think it is a problem. For instance, one might say that if a chemical causes cancer in one in a million people, then it is bad. Furthermore, information about hazards comes from experiments on nonhuman animals and natural experiments (which is an epidemiological term for catastrophes) on people.

To put hazard identification in context, then, scientists studying the cancerous effects of chemicals in food are asked to look for the ten-year-old cause of a proliferation of cells in one in a million bodies. One needs either to sacrifice a million animals or to watch a million people exposed to the chemical that might (or might not) be a problem for ten years.

One could be forgiven for thinking the whole exercise quixotic. How do investigators get around this problem? On the animal side, you can give various high doses to fewer animals and then connect the dots and try to estimate what would happen at low doses. But is it a straight line? If it causes cancer in 50 percent of the rats at one dose and in 25 percent of the rats at half that dose, does it cause cancer in five in a million at one-ten millionth of the dose? Is everything toxic only less so the less of it one eats? Or are some things good for people up to a point (a "threshold"), and then they become poisonous? Everybody knows that, for some things, like strychnine, salt, and potatoes, small amounts can stimulate and large amounts can kill. But is that true for everything?

If something causes cancer in rats at high doses, will it cause cancer in people at low doses? Now scientists not only are making an inference from high to low doses but are jumping across species. Looking at natural disasters and natural exposures is helpful, but only for those chemicals that are already out there being used. For chemicals that aren't on the market, scientists try to combine information from animals, from effects on bacteria, and from their basic knowledge of chemistry: does this new chemical look like anything else we know?

One can see why, in the United States, legislators put in a law, the Delaney Clause, which says that there should not be anything in food that causes cancer at any level in any animal.

It is a kind of safety-in-abstinence theory. But is it realistic? Is it any wonder that scientists quarrel about these things? After all, some people's lives and other people's livelihoods may be at stake. What is worth more—your job at fifty, or my not having cancer at seventy? This process is value laden right from the start.

The International Agency for Research on Cancer (IARC) reviews various pieces of information from all over the world about cancer and chemicals and tries to group them according to the following criteria: (1) the agent is carcinogenic to humans, (2) the agent is probably carcinogenic to humans, (3) the agent is possibly carcinogenic to humans, (4) the agent is not classifiable as to its carcinogenicity to humans, and (5) the agent is probably not carcinogenic to humans.

These are judgments, based on the best evidence available. They do not include consideration of outcomes other than cancer. And they do not take seriously the fact that every human being has a unique history and a unique sensitivity, or resistance, to each chemical. This is statistical probability at its scariest, and it is probably the best we can do under the circumstances.

For many effects other than cancer, scientists estimate thresholds (No Observed Effect Levels, or NOELs) based on animal data, throw in a safety factor of 100, and call it an Acceptable Daily Intake. International agencies such as the World Health Organization define acceptable daily intake as an "estimate of the amount of a substance in food or drinking water, expressed on a body-weight basis, that can be ingested over a lifetime without appreciable risk." The word "acceptable" is an unfortunate choice, since the consumers of these chemicals have not agreed to any level of consumption. The Environmental Protection organization in the United States calls it, perhaps more accurately, a Reference Dose. It is a level at which scientists guess that politicians ought to do something.

Having determined some level of hazard for a chemical, someone needs to figure out whether or not people are being exposed to this chemical at a level that might hurt them. The World Health Organization has produced guidelines for calculating this exposure level with varying degrees of precision. One option is to determine what levels of residues might occur in foods if "good agricultural practices" (their words, not mine) are followed. Then some poor bureaucrat, stuck with the thankless task of developing regulations, can guess what an average person might eat and from that guess how much of which chemicals they are exposed to. This step assumes that all farmers use the chemical and that all edible parts of the crop attain a certain level of residue.

One can take this a step further and actually test what is in crops, meat, milk, and eggs. Most countries do this, at least with some of the food. You cannot test all of the food, or there would not be any left for anyone to eat. Furthermore, you can't always be sure that the particular type or form of the chemical for which you are testing is one that is there, or is the one that might cause problems. And finally, this process does not account for the effects of food preparation like cooking or peeling.

Some countries, such as the United States and Canada, have enough money to conduct what are called market basket, or total diet, studies. Investigators are sent out to supermarkets to buy a "market basket" full of what are considered typical foods eaten by an average family. The foods are then sent to laboratories, where they are prepared in a way that is considered typical, or average, for that food. Finally, the foods thus prepared are tested in the laboratory for a range of possibly toxic substances.

A myriad of questions arise. Which average family? What is normal? Which farms did the food come from? If governments have endless money and endless time, they can test all of the foods in every possible diet and then perhaps manufacture a little gizmo that will spit out a daily human-made chemical-intake measure. Is it worth it? Will people be better and healthier for it? Will the planet be a better place to live? But I am getting beyond myself. What I am talking about here is exposure.

Another way to determine exposure is to measure what people have in their bodies at any given time. Some studies have examined residues in breast milk and fatty tissue, blood, hair, and nails. That will work for chemicals with long lives in our bodies, such as PCBs and DDT, but not for the hit-and-run type of chemical. Furthermore, while the information is helpful (or would be if it were collected in a more rational way), it still does not tell us what those chemicals might be doing in our naturally deteriorating bodies.

This brings us to the fourth step in risk assessment, risk characterization, where scientists try to put all this information together. After they have decided what the hazard of a chemical might be, and estimated how much some people might be exposed to, they still need to determine its effects in the "real world." What proportion of which groups of people are being exposed to how much chemical, and what is happening to their bodies? Perhaps the chemicals are just sitting there, not doing anything, waiting for us to die so that they can get on with their lives in the wider world. Maybe they are thinking about causing cancer.

In addition, biological scientists find themselves ill equipped to deal with the social components of risk and the value-laden decisions that are inherent in managing that risk. Hence they walk about, fingering their microbiological rosaries, repeating things like "Our food supply is the safest in the world," as if the repetition of this litany will somehow make things right.

After risks are characterized using risk assessment, the activities shift to risk management, when governments try to use risk assessment to make decisions. This stage is closely related to risk communication, which is either a public discussion about risks, such as the one I am engaging in here, and which I encourage in my classes, or a series of lectures to an ignorant public from people who think they have all the answers.

If risk assessment appears to be a house of cards built in a sandbox just before a thundershower, then risk management and risk communication consist of a bunch of grownups convincing the rest of us kids that the house of cards is really the Empire State Building. Scientists, government regulators, consumer advocates, and industry spokespeople are not very good at understanding and communicating the inherent uncertainty in what is known, what the options for action are, and what the consequences of those actions might be. Some still act as if the effects of chemicals can and should be proven in some absolute sense before they are regulated. It should be clear from the foregoing, however, that even if everyone knew everything about all the chemicals that our best scientists knew, we would still be squabbling.

Some people try to differentiate "real risk" from "perceived risk," usually with the idea of discrediting you because they know what is real and you only perceive things. The distinction is usually specious. It is true that the dangers you think are there are not always there, but it is also true that the dangers they "know" are there are already strained through a sieve of value judgments about what is valuable in this society, what kinds of risks are worth taking, and who should bear those risks for whose benefit.

One thing that has puzzled regulators and scientists is that public anxiety seems to be increasing even as our technical scientific knowledge expands and our apparent certainty increases. This trend has led to a great deal of anxiety among regulators and industrial representatives. How can one make the public see that there is no problem? How can one allay their fears?

Some of this puzzlement occurs because public debate is not very good at separating out population phenomena, such as the very low rates of disease attributable to foodborne chemicals, from individual phenomena—that is, the fact that you or I might get sick or die from a particular exposure. This lack of differentiation between levels of concern is a phenomenon familiar to epidemiologists but is not as commonly understood even by other scientists. Every case of disease may be a cause of anguish to the people involved, but not every case of disease is of public health importance. In fact, paying equal attention to every case of disease can be a way of undermining public health, as resources are set aside to deal with rare, albeit serious (and to medical specialists therefore interesting) diseases.

Risk communication is part of a public conversation based on all the available knowledge. It is a political and moral debate based on a variety of evidence. As a society, we need democratic discussion and arguments about what we value and ways of assessing the quality of information we are using. The furor over the chemical Alar in the 1980s illustrates many of these points.

In March 1989, out of concern about a chemical with the trade name Alar, schools in New York and Los Angeles pulled apples from their cafeterias. The chemical that caused this concern was daminozide, a substance used to promote color and uniform ripening in several fruits, including apples. This decision was accompanied by a drop in apple sales across North America and assurances by various levels of government that apples were safe. The chemical and apple industries denounced irrational consumers and blamed the media for a "disinformation scare." A closer look at this episode elucidates how risk assessment has been dealt with publicly.

In 1984, the United States Environmental Protection Agency (EPA) announced it was reviewing its risk assessment of daminozide and its breakdown product UDMH (Unsymmetrical Dimethyl Hydrazine), originally based on high-dose studies done on rats and mice in the 1970s. In January 1985, this assessment estimated one extra cancer death per ten thousand individuals exposed to Alar. The EPA proposed a ban on the substance. After receiving criticism from the industry and meeting with consumers and other branches of government, the

EPA lowered the acceptable residue level and asked the manufacturer, Uniroyal, to conduct more studies. A flurry of activities by various state governments, consumer groups, and industry interests followed. Several states petitioned the EPA to ban Alar, Ralph Nader filed a lawsuit, supermarkets and food processors announced a boycott, and apple growers announced a voluntary ban. In 1988, Alar residues were found on apples advertised as being free of the substance.

In February 1989, the EPA said its new studies suggested that Alar posed an unacceptable cancer risk of 3.5 per 100,000 persons and asked Uniroyal to voluntarily withdraw it from the market. The company declined to do so. On February 26, 60 *Minutes* aired a program on Alar and talked to scientists and politicians who, in turn, talked about children dying on cancer wards. The day after this program, the Natural Resources Defense Council (NRDC) released the report that had been used by 60 *Minutes*, which estimated a risk of 2.4 cancers per 10,000 persons. Public debate and controversy raged across North America until June 1989, when Uniroyal voluntarily halted sales.

Although industry people blamed the 60 *Minutes* program and the NRDC "disinformation" for economic difficulties among apple growers, a study of apple sales in New York by Michigan State University economists Eileen van Ravensway and John Hoehn gave a slightly different picture. Apple sales began declining as early as the 1984 EPA announcement and continued to fall, with a drop (though not a statistically significant one) after the 60 *Minutes* show. In short, consumers acted in a reasonable fashion to messages about risk they were receiving from scientific authorities. They were not irrational or fanatical.

At the same time, the media and politicians did manipulate the facts to their advantage. One politician talked about looking at the poor kids on the cancer wards and then asking whether you still wanted Alar. This statement either was based on ignorance or was the crassest form of abuse of children's suffering. While both the EPA and the NRDC based their estimates on exposure to apples in childhood (though they differed on quantities), the risk estimates they calculated, like most risk assessment estimates, were for cases of cancer over a lifetime. Somewhere between thirty-five and two hundred and forty American children exposed to daminozide might develop cancer over the course of a lifetime, depending largely on what their other life experiences are. Although this might still be an unacceptable level, one might question whether it was an appropriate dragon to be slaying, given that overeating fatty fast foods, suicides, sexually transmitted diseases, and car accidents will kill many more children.

Several authors have used tables and graphs that they say compare "actual risks" with "perceived risks." These comparisons are often of more emotional than scientific value, however. In one comparison, the high risks associated with getting injured while bicycle riding are compared with the estimated low risks associated with ingesting pesticides. But thirty years of riding a bike is good for both me and the planet. Is thirty years of eating pesticides? Other writers have compared the high risks of cancer from natural toxins in food with the small risks associated with manufactured chemicals. Are we to conclude that because aflatoxins are worse than many manufactured chemicals, we should not worry about the manufactured varieties of toxins? It seems to be a poor basis for public policy to justify one bad thing by pointing to another. Maybe we should screen traditional foods for natural carcinogens and seek ways to (1) warn people that these carcinogens are present and might pose a risk, (2) modify storage and shipment procedures so as to reduce the presence of, say, aflatoxins, and (3) breed plant varieties that lack the toxic component.

In some published comparisons, the "actual" risks reflect the probability that insurance companies will have to pay a claim for negative outcomes from such events as motor vehicle accidents or accidental pesticide poisoning. Given the many factors in our diet and lifestyle that contribute to heart disease or cancer, and the long time lag between our bad habits and their natural consequences, I would be surprised if insurance companies see many claims against specific chronic chemical exposures.

What the "perceived" risks refer to is not clear. Do people rank risks based on the chance of accidental death or the possibility of cancer or immunological and reproductive effects in their children after forty years of continuous exposure? Or do they differentiate between risks freely chosen (such as skydiving and bungee jumping) and risks imposed by others (for the others' profit)? It is not a trivial distinction.

Estimating the reduction in life expectancy has been proposed as one way to rank risks. Because cancer tends to occur late in life, it is not at the top of the list. Diet-related cancer would not be considered very serious according to this criterion of ranking. Heart disease, being single, and cigarette smoking are at the top of that list. North Americans are conditioned to value their freedom to take even very high risks, and it is not surprising that we would choose to commit more public money, for less effect, to reduce risks perceived to be imposed by someone else.

How do we deal with chemical risks in the context of this uncertainty? Some people have responded by looking at, say, total diet studies, determining which foods are more likely to have residues, and avoiding them. That is the save-your-soul-and-damn-the-world approach. I can save you the trouble of poisoning your mind with endless books about poisons in food. In short, fatty foods are more likely to contain fat-soluble chemicals, which include most of the pesticides and industrial chemicals we are worried about. Beyond that, we are on shaky ground. Organic foods have fewer chemicals and are better for the environment than nonorganic foods, but they are just as likely to harbor infectious agents or parasites. And are mass-produced organic foods that are then shipped over long distances better than locally produced foods that use some chemicals? I think not.

One could say that just to be safe, there should not be any extraneous chemicals in our food, that the only poisons present should be those produced by members of the ecosystem other than ourselves. Food industry people will argue that our tests are getting so good, industrial and agricultural chemicals are so ubiquitous, and the levels of chemicals being detected are so small that this approach is ludicrous. To the extent that we are being led by the nose by our testing technology, I have to agree with them. Our society should not let our tests make our decisions for us.

At the same time, one can make a convincing case for a general policy of avoiding all residues in food. Trace amounts of antibiotics in milk may not be doing any damage to me, but I do not want them there any more than I want a fly (also harmless) in my soup. This brings me back to one of my recurring themes: that the most important questions are about values.

Some may suggest that the presence of chemicals such as pesticides in our food is a necessary side effect of our abundant food supply. But first, such a cost-benefit analysis overlooks the fact that those who reap the greatest benefit from this food supply are not the people who are paying the cost. Second, it is not clear that the equation is as obvious as has been suggested. Several researchers, including David Pimental and his colleagues at Cornell University, have concluded that humanity would not starve if pesticides were withdrawn. A few crops would suffer, at least in the short run, but a shift to fewer pesticides and fertilizers might get humanity out of this rut of promoting good bookkeeping and sloppy biology down on the farm.

If our society did want to reduce dependence (through fertilizers, pesticides, and long-distance travel) on fossil-fuel based inputs, how would we do it? Regulation is necessary to protect public safety but will not cure our addiction to manufactured chemicals. Controlling chemicals on some farms may run up against the same individual-rights bias that motivates other farmers not to use any chemicals at all. Another approach to this problem is for consumers to work directly with local farmers. If you know the general geographical area and have some knowledge of the regulations that govern agriculture there, or better yet, if you know the farmers, then you have some idea what might be in the food they produce, and perhaps have some influence over which foods are grown. Eating locally can have global implications. It provides an opportunity to peek out from behind your blindfold before you get into bed with that tomato or hunk of meat. The farmer, knowing you as a consumer of his or her environment, will sleep more easily knowing there is a market for the farm's produce. My ideal food is locally grown and organic, but if I have to choose between them, I'll pick locally grown.

I still eat imported food, but I view that practice as a luxury rather than a right.

Risk assessment is an important way of organizing our information about chemicals and the risks they pose, but it is not a panacea. It is a kind of Hamburger Helper for those whom we have delegated to cook up our regulations and enforce them. It is a way of organizing some very messy information about chronic exposures to chemicals from a variety of sources and setting up rules for making decisions and setting policies. But it's not the only option.

Instead of using risk assessment to guess what might happen, we could start at the other end of the equation, with cases of illness, and work back to guess what proportion might be from foodborne chemical contamination. There are hundreds of thousands of cases of cancer reported in North America every year, and only a small proportion of those are from exposures through food, while there are millions of cases of foodborne diseases. Still, if somebody gave me the choice between a high probability of getting diarrhea and a small probability of getting cancer, I confess I'd stock up on chicken soup, flat ginger ale, and bananas, and head for the bathroom. While I was sitting there, I'd think about danger and risk and see if there might be another way to come at this problem. I'll return to the topic in chapter 14, after we've mulled over a few of the messy problems that risk analysis was supposed to solve.

10

ONE PERSON'S CURE, ANOTHER PERSON'S COFFIN

ANTIBACTERIALS, PESTICIDES, AND PRESERVATIVES

S O YOU WANT to grow lots of wholesome food, undamaged by fungi or insects? You want to prevent suffering and death in millions of people and animals? You want to save tons of food from spoiling, food that could be used to feed hungry people the world over, food that, if it does spoil, will have to be replaced, thus putting greater, potentially environmentally destructive demands on farmers? Welcome to the world of pesticides, antibacterial drugs, and preservatives.

The motivation to produce these chemicals is much more complex than that. It includes greed and power and all the usual frailties that masquerade as wisdom and philanthropy. But underlying the normal human vices are the more lofty goals I have stated. Does that mean we are stuck with agricultural chemicals? Are there no alternatives? The people who make their living selling the chemicals will tell you that the alternatives are utopian or ignorant, but they have a vested interest in keeping things as they are. There *are* intelligent alternatives; we *can* learn from history.

An antibacterial drug is a chemical that works against bacteria, either by killing them or by stopping them from multiplying. Antibacterials include both mineral-based chemicals, such as sulfa drugs, and antibiotics. Antibiotics are antibacterial drugs that are naturally produced by living things, usually fungi. They include some of our most common chemicals, like tetracycline and penicillin. In using them, we are simply carrying on a long evolutionary tradition of producing substances that help us to stay alive. In that, at least, we are not different from the black mold in the leftover yogurt at the back of the refrigerator.

The world market for antibacterial drugs is in the tens of billions of dollars (U.S.). These drugs have come a long way from the early part of the twentieth century, when they were viewed by many as a utopian dream. Today we hardly realize how miraculous their discovery was, how many millions of lives they have saved. Like prodigal children, we have taken this precious inheritance for granted, and squandered it, and we may yet live to regret it.

In a talk he gave in Australia in the summer of 2006, Peter Daszak, executive director of the Consortium for Conservation Medicine, highlighted Western Europe and the northeastern United States as major hot spots for emerging infectious diseases. When some of us in the room expressed surprise at this news, having been conditioned by media reports to think of Southeast Asia as the most worrisome spot on the planet, he pointed out that many of the most serious emerging infections were antibacterial-resistant strains of bacteria. And these bacteria were appearing where antibacterial drugs had been used most intensely.

When I wrote the first edition of this book, in 1991, antibacterial resistance was considered important scientifically, but the "resistance sceptics," much like those who claimed that cigarettes were nonaddictive, or those who claim that global warming is a controversial issue among scientists (it is not), seemed to hold the public's attention. Today antimicrobial resistance is considered one of the most important medical issues in the world. Governments in North America, Europe, and elsewhere have begun to mount campaigns to bring it under control. And the industries that benefit from widespread and reckless use of these valuable drugs have mounted a stiff rearguard action that confuses strong, unsubstantiated opinions with genuine scientific skepticism.

In the early days, it was suggested that one might wish to add antibacterial drugs deliberately to our food. After all, did they not kill bacteria? Do not bacteria make us sick? Could not low doses in the milk help to prevent sickness in people? Scientists have learned a few things since those heady days in the mid-1900s, although many agriculturalists still argue in favor of adding antibacterial drugs to animal feeds to promote growth. About 40 percent of U.S. sales of antibacterial drugs are destined for use in animals. A person would have to be pretty naive or wilfully iniquitous not to expect at least some of these drugs to return to us in the form of resistant bacterial populations and food residues.

Antibacterial residues in food can, in rare instances, be directly toxic to people or be involved in the development of allergies. From a public health point of view, these are not the most important negative outcomes of using antimicrobial drugs in agriculture. For the dairy industry, the fact that antibacterial residues in milk interfere with starter cultures for fermented food products such as cheese, buttermilk, and yogurt is of immense importance economically. When looking at the overall food system, however, the greatest impact of the profligate use of antibacterial drugs in agriculture (such as in animal feeds) is the development of antibacterial-resistant strains of bacteria in animals and people. As a result, when veterinarians or physicians confront serious diseases, the best treatments are not available to them. More people infected with drug-resistant strains of bacteria have been hospitalized and died than people infected with strains of the same bacteria that are susceptible to drugs. The multiple-antibiotic resistant *Salmonella typhimurium* DT104 and Methicillin-resistant *Staphylococcus aureus* (MRSA) covered in earlier chapters are but the latest manifestations of a problem that scientists have been aware of for more than a quarter century.

In 1985, the Los Angeles County Health Department laboratory noted a big increase (to 298, from 69 the previous year) in reports of people getting sick from infection with a particular strain of *Salmonella*—*S. Newport,* of folk festival fame. One peculiarity of these bacteria was that they clutched within them, like a spy's microchip, a precious little plasmid, a tiny bit of DNA not attached to the main gene of the bacterium. In this way, the information in the plasmid could be shared among friendly bacteria during their social intercourse without compromising their essential being. The valuable (to the bacteria) information in this plasmid contained codes for resistance to several antibacterial drugs, including one of the most effective (and possibly dangerous) ones we have—chloramphenicol.

In one of those fourteen-author medical reports for which the *New England Journal of Medicine* is famous, investigators described their search for the origins, not just of the *Salmonella,* but of the resistance plasmid it carried. They studied people who had the infection and compared them with those who did not. They stuck their noses into people's dietary habits. They cultured suspect foods from suspect sources. They swabbed the slaughterhouses and poked around in cow manure on California dairy farms. This is the sort of thing public health investigators are expected to do.

The study came up with two kinds of behavior that put people at risk for infection: taking antibiotics (which the antibiotic-resistant bacteria consider a welcome subsidy) and eating hamburger or raw meat. They tracked down the hamburger from a couple of implicated restaurants to one particular factory that specialized in removing bones from meat. From there they went back to the abattoir where the cows had been killed. The farther the investigators got away from the people who got sick, the cooler and more tangled the trail became. They followed it through auction houses, sales barns, and trucks until they were standing out on a highway looking at the still slightly steaming trail of cow manure. The trail led out to the dairy farm community that provided the old cows that became the hamburger. Dairy farmers, on the advice of my fellow veterinarians, were using chloramphenicol (never licensed for use in food animals in the United States but always very effective). Some of the old cows did not respond well to their treatment, and sick and stressed (and probably shedding *Salmonella*), they made their way on to the tables and into the bodies of the people of Los Angeles.

Some veterinarians and agriculturalists disputed the conclusions of the Los Angeles investigation, resonating, as they do, with the *Just So* stories of Rudyard Kipling (for example, "How the Elephant Got His Nose"). But really, should anyone be surprised? It's basic Biology 101. Bacterial survivors tend to be resistant to the drugs that they are challenged with over a period of time. Not only that, and perhaps more of a problem, is that if you give, say, penicillin, the bacteria will develop resistance not only to penicillin but probably to several other drugs as well. Scientists have known about this kind of linked resistance for a long time as well. Behaviors, in microbes as much as in people, tend to come in clusters. Since bacteria often make the move from life in the rural gut worlds of animals to the high city life of the human intestine, it would be silly to suppose that the resistant bacteria in animals would not, at least some of the time, cause disease in people.

The conclusions drawn from the investigation were based on a mixture of science and sleuthing that is the hallmark of great epidemic investigations. Chloramphenicol is rarely used in humans (meaning use of the drug in humans was an unlikely source of resistance), and the conclusions, while not proof in a scientific sense, certainly gain high marks in the annals of common sense.

Supporters of the use of antibacterial drugs in animal feeds argue that the antibacterial resistance problems in people are caused by overuse of these drugs by physicians; antibacterial resistance in livestock is the result of overzealous treatments by veterinarians. This notion betrays a complete lack of understanding of bacterial ecology and the complexity of biological movement in industrial agriculture.

More contentious is the discussion about the economic benefits of subtherapeutic levels of antibiotics in feed versus the risks associated with this practice. It may be true that this practice has enabled farmers to keep animals in close confinement, get more growth with less feed (increase their feed efficiency), and hence to use less land to greater benefit. However, most of the major costs of this method of agriculture—general bacterial contamination of the environment and water supplies, antibacterial resistance—have been foisted onto the general public and onto future generations. Some of us who have children are not happy with this trade-off. Bacteria are now developing resistance to some of the "drugs of last resort," the ones used in people when all the others fail; much of this resistance stems from the use of related drugs in animal agriculture.

Historically, several families of drugs have been used widely enough in the agriculture and food system to be of broad public health concern: the tetracyclines, the penicillin family, chloramphenicol, and sulfonamides.

Tetracyclines are among the most widely used antibiotics worldwide. They are used to treat many infections in people, though rarely in children, since they bind to bones and teeth and cause "browning." They are also used to treat many animal diseases and have been the antibiotics of choice for animal feed manufacturers who include them to promote quicker growth and greater feed efficiency in chickens and pigs. They have been injected into oral rabies vaccine baits so that biologists can tell which foxes have taken up the vaccine. As the result of this widespread use, they sometimes show up as residues in food. More worrisome is that bacteria are being selected that are resistant not only to tetracycline but to several other antibiotics. Fortunately, from a public health viewpoint, even low levels of tetracycline in milk affect the quality of yogurt, so the dairy industry tends to regulate tetracycline use even without government intervention. In this instance, at least, the creameries and the health officials are fighting the same battle.

Penicillins (there is a whole family of them) are considered to be some of the least toxic, most beneficial drugs we know. In the last couple of decades, the main problem, besides bacterial resistance, is that people can develop allergies to them. Estimates vary from 4 to 15 allergic reactions per 100,000 members of the population to 1 fatal reaction in 67,000 courses of treatment to 1 to 5 in 10,000 courses. The Joint FAO/WHO Expert Committee on Food Additives (JECFA) of the World Health Organization has suggested that somewhere between 3 and 10 percent of all people are allergic to penicillins. How much of this is because of food exposure we cannot say, though from a public health viewpoint, one could argue that none of it should be.

Severe reactions to penicillin in foods are not often reported. In one case, a child in the United States was said to have died of a heart attack after eating cat food; the level of penicillin in the cat food was more than six hundred times the allowable limit in beef destined for human consumption. There are no regulated limits to residues in pet foods. As in many case reports of allergic reactions to residues in food, the physicians were not able to differentiate between a reaction to the residue and one to the food itself.

It is legitimate to ask why there is penicillin in cat food. Are farmers using too many antibiotics? Do too many animals get sick because of the way they are raised? Should ecological efficiency, which dictates that animals not fit for human consumption be fed to dogs and cats, be allowed to put at risk children who might get into pet dishes? One could just as easily ask why a child is eating cat food. What were the social causes of the child's death? A poor family on welfare? A naive relationship between pets and people? A failure of public health education?

Most reactions attributed to penicillin in food are less dramatic than death; skin rashes are more likely to occur at the low doses of exposure that one might encounter through food.

The use of tetracyclines in food may lead to drug resistance, and the use of pencillin may cause allergic reactions, but chloramphenicol is toxic. Chloramphenicol is an antibiotic that has periodically stirred the political pot over the last thirty years. Although it was never licensed for use in food animals in the United States and was banned in Canada in the mid-1980s, scientists still periodically detect it, or its effects, in various foods, the Los Angeles epidemic being a case in point.

Chloramphenicol has been used in animals because it has been effective against many serious diseases, because of resistance to other antibiotics, and because adverse toxic reactions in animals have not often been reported. My own work in the early 1980s demonstrated that chloramphenicol was the most frequently used antibiotic in dairy calves in Ontario. It was used by such environmentally and socially conscious veterinarians as the author of this book. I did not know then what I know now. The International Agency for Research on Cancer says chloramphenicol may be carcinogenic to humans. Hazards of chloramphenicol related to *clinical* use in people have included an irreversible destruction of the cells that produce red blood cells (aplastic anemia). The cases that have been reported invariably occur after treatment, rather than from exposure through food. Because this condition occurs in children and (to spite the toxicologists) does not appear to be related to dose levels, public health officials want to see this chemical kept under severe restrictions, with no "acceptable" safe limits set by the World Health Organization.

The sulfa drugs also raise a concern beyond those of toxicity and allergy—that of environmental persistence. Adverse reactions, such as skin rashes, anemia, and thyroid dysfunctions, have been reported for therapeutic doses of sulfa drugs, but those are not what scientists are concerned about when they look at food. They want to know whether the drugs cause cancer. Scientists who have reviewed the literature say there is not enough information to make a decision on the matter. What is known is that sulfa residues have been a continuing problem in a significant percentage of pigs (particularly so-called barbecue pigs) marketed in the United States and Canada, as well as in "bob veal" calves (calves fed primarily a milk-based diet and sold at less than 150 pounds).

Aside from their use in feeds, antibacterial drugs are used to cure sick animals. If a farmer has a sick cow, the cheapest, most convenient way to get that animal back growing or producing milk is often to give it a shot of antibiotic. Since consumers demand cheap food, farmers—with a great deal of egging on and support by chemical companies, to be sure—have responded by making efficiency the bottom line.

Crowding animals together, which promotes the spread of disease, is more economically efficient than not crowding them, especially if antibacterial drugs are used. To get the most out of the animal—say, a milk cow—the farmer tries to get the milk from a sick cow back into the system as quickly as possible. Rules have been set to manage this process. Each drug in each licensed species has a withdrawal time, which is the amount of time the farmer must wait before putting the milk or meat into the human food chain. But withdrawal times do not apply to doses not recommended on the label or to unlicensed drugs. Farmers do not want to see an animal suffer from disease, but they don't want to lose the money on the emotional invest-ment that animal represents either. What to do? Try unlicensed drugs? Try licensed drugs at higher doses? How long to wait?

No one knows. In the meantime, scientific researchers in the United States have developed some tests that can detect minute amounts of drug residues in meat and milk. One test made front-page headlines in the United States and Canada in the 1980s by detecting chloramphenicol, tetracyclines, penicil-lin, and sulfa drugs in the commercial milk supply. What does this mean? Whom do we blame? Some scientists argue that at the levels being detected, the tests could be picking up natu-ral antibiotics or antibioticlike substances being produced by the fungi and other plants that live all around us. Some dairies that pick the milk up from the farms test the milk using the new tests and, if antibacterial drugs are detected, penalize the farmer in some fashion (by dumping the milk and not paying for it, for instance).

Some farmers are welcoming a spate of new cow-side tests so that they can check their milk before selling it. Other farm-ers are turning to alternatives, substituting, for instance, homeo-pathic remedies for antibacterial drugs.

Urban consumers need to rethink the demand for cheap food and support farmers in their efforts to make our food safe. So far, city dwellers have not been much good at help-ing farmers make the transition to organic methods and bio-regional marketing (selling food as locally as possible—that is, within a given ecologically defined area). In part this is because farmers have been manipulated into a corner by chemical companies and agrifood industries that like to pretend they are in the farming game.

Those of us who would like to see changes in farming practices should have no illusions. Agribusiness owners are city people in the business of making money. Helping farmers does not make money. Even as information about spreading resistance to the old drugs like tetracycline and penicillin has appeared, companies have quietly introduced new drugs to take their place. New drugs are a good thing, but unfortunately, they have found their way into the agricultural feed market almost as quickly as into the hospitals. Physicians are now reporting resistance to vancomycin, related to avoparcin used in animals, and synercid, related to virginiamycin, which is used in chickens.

There are some rays of hope. The prevalence and amount of antibacterial residues in milk in the industrialized world have decreased in the last thirty years. There are even some people who are testing the tests to see what they really detect, and a small bit of research is going on to find less stressful ways of rearing animals that require fewer, or no, antibacterial drugs. Still, there is almost no research being published about the alternative remedies.

It is reasonable, sensible, and scientifically grounded to ban the use of antibacterial drugs as growth promoters in animals. Sweden did so in 1986, as did Danish chicken and pig farmers in the late 1990s. The Danes and the Swedes, as far as I can tell, don't seem to be suffering unduly. On January 1, 2006, the European Union countries as a group followed suit. North American regulators of these things, who have not yet acted as decisively, seem to have a more Hollywood-ish voodoo approach to these matters, but that might be seen as a denigration of the vodun religion, which has more merit and legitimacy than this waste of medically important drugs. To their credit, some companies, such as McDonald's Corporation, will buy chicken only from producers that do not use antibiotics for routine disease prevention, and some of the larger poultry producers have followed suit.

Not only do we need to ban the use of antibacterial drugs as growth promoters, but we need to more tightly control therapeutic uses of antibacterial drugs. In some countries, they are available only through pharmacists on prescription from veterinarians. Physicians already do this. It should not take a great leap of imagination to extend this practice to all species. Consumers need to be aware that farmers do not want to see residues in our food supply; this is not a rural plot against arrogant city slickers.

One unanswered question is what to do with animal carcasses that contain antibacterial residues. Bury them? That seems a waste. Make them into pet food, as we do now? The agrifood business has always been way ahead of urban environmentalists in recycling. But recycling in a system where residues and pollutants occur is a dangerous game. In words attributed to the poet Federico Garcia Lorca, "Life is not a dream. Careful! Careful! Careful!"

The use of hormonal substances in food-producing animals brings home perhaps most strongly both the public fears around food safety and the true nature of the debate taking place. As in all areas of food safety, it is easy to get lost among all the names and lose sight of the overall nature of the problem we are dealing with. It's worth mentioning three substances specifically, however. Like most of the chemicals used in our food supply, some of these are natural and some are imitations of natural.

Since the 1950s, hormones have been used to promote growth in cattle. By and large, the people who sell them and use them have argued that they enable us to increase growth rates and feed efficiency. These, in turn, make farmers more

economically competitive and farming more ecologically sustainable (by using less land to support the same number of
animals). In this respect, the basic arguments about diethylstil-
bestrol (DES), used to make cattle grow faster on less food, and
bovine somatotrophin (BST), used to make them give more milk,
are not much different.

The way DES was mishandled generated a storm among scientists, drug sellers (pharmaceutical companies), and drug users
(the public) that we have yet to learn from. A full consideration
of all its ramifications is well beyond what can be covered in a
general book like this, but a few insights should be underlined.
Approved for human use in the United States in 1947, to prevent miscarriages, it very quickly became widely used for a host
of unrelated purposes, some of which only became apparent to
the public when the drug was banned. It was banned for use in
lambs and chickens in 1959 and from cattle feed in 1980.

Yet from the 1940s on, there was medical evidence that DES
caused cancers in a variety of animals, including people. Each
government department, each scientific discipline, each public
interest group was so narrowly focused on one particular outcome (promoting animal growth, preventing miscarriages), usually one that benefited the members of that group, that they
refused to even admit that there was a world beyond their blink-
ered vision, that every benefit came with a cost, and that actions
in one part of the ecosystem might have effects elsewhere.
Throw into this mix the usual hucksters, civic-minded but conservative regulators, naive promisers of chemical solutions to all
human problems, scientific reductionists, and just plain opportunists, and you have a messy situation that has since plagued
all risk assessments of hormone use.

The DES controversy has colored all subsequent debate about
the use of hormones, whether naturally occurring or synthetic
(sometimes referred to as xenobiotic). All scientists are now sus-

pect, as are all hormones, and no reassurances can help that. Outbreaks of premature sexual development in children in Italy and Puerto Rico have been ascribed to sexual hormones in the meat, though none was ever found, and other explanations were available. The burden now falls on those who want to introduce new substances to prove that they are safe, rather than on the public and its academic allies to demonstrate that they cause harm. This change has occurred in an environment in which scientists are under increasing pressure, because of government cutbacks to research and education, to commercialize their findings. While the changing nature of this debate has been the subject of much academic argument, the general public is often left in the dark. What kinds of trade-offs are we making? Whose benefits outweigh whose harm?

Many consumers are quick to attribute ill health to something in food, and sometimes they are right, even if the evidence is very shaky. There is always a probability of food contamination. Although the DES debate is rooted in concern about public health, the continuing fight about the use of bovine somatotrophin (BST, sometimes called bovine growth hormone), has more to do with politics, economics, and value systems. The public health impacts are there, but they are more systemically complex. Does our society really need more milk production? What are the benefits? How does it affect water and land use? Cows that produce more milk are more likely to get mastitis, because of the stress on their udders, which means that they are more likely to get treated with antibacterial drugs. And scientists already know where that road leads—to more antibacterial-resistant bacteria. There may be good health and ecological reasons for increasing the production of milk, but these need to be considered in a context of systemic trade-offs. Are there limits to good things, such as producing milk (or even saving individual lives through medical interventions)? If so, what are they? Who is debating this? Who decides on the limits? And, as ·Katharine Farrell, one of my younger colleagues, asked in her PhD thesis: who decides who decides?

One of the more interesting hormonal-type substances to hit the agricultural market in the past decade is something called clenbuterol, which is used for increasing the proportion of muscle in carcasses (resulting in leaner meat). Reports of illegal use of the drug have come from both North America and Europe. In 1990, 125 people in Spain were hospitalized with increased heart rate, muscle tremors, headache, dizziness, fever, and chills. Epidemiologists traced the cause of the epidemic to beef liver containing very high levels of the drug. It appeared that the farmer may have overdosed his animals and then slaughtered them for meat to get some of his money out of them before they died.

The use of clenbuterol is apparently a response to consumer demands for leaner meat. It is also used by bodybuilders and dieters to increase their lean muscle mass. When we demand something from farmers, do we know what we are asking?

If antibacterial drugs and injected, manufactured hormones appear to be a special concern of meat eaters, pesticides are indiscriminate.

ON SATURDAY, June 29, 1985, six people from two families in Oregon got together for some striped watermelon. The big U.S. holiday weekend was coming up. The melon tasted fine. Half an hour after their meal, five of the attendees suffered nausea, vomiting, abdominal pain, diarrhea, blurred vision, muscle twitching, slurred speech, and an odd sensation around the lips and tongue. The one person who was not sick had not eaten any watermelon. They all got better within four hours without any treatment. The health department considered tampering or pesticide poisoning as a possibility. Tampering seemed unlikely, however, and no carbamates or organophosphates, the two most likely pesticides, could be detected in the piece of melon that remained.

Two days later, on July 1, two more people showed up at an emergency room with similar symptoms. The doctors who saw them, unaware of the incident on June 29, diagnosed an intestinal infection, sent the patients home, and duly reported this occurrence to the health unit the next day. The Oregon State Public Health Division alerted five local area hospitals and contacted the U.S. Food and Drug Administration in California and Washington State. There were no other reports of similar illnesses. Still, officials were nervous. The Fourth of July, the time of greatest per capita watermelon consumption in the United States, was just around the corner. The possibility of widespread poisoning was high, but a recall could devastate the growers and, if later proven to be unjustified, put the health officials in the legal hot seat.

On the morning of July 3, another family of six reported getting sick after eating striped watermelon. Immediately, health officials held a press conference, putting out a health advisory and alerting local health departments and emergency rooms around the state. The distributor voluntarily recalled its striped watermelons. The pesticide aldicarb was detected in the fruit eaten by the July 3 family. California instituted a program whereby watermelons were stickered if they came from farms where growers signed affidavits that they had not used aldicarb in their fields for twelve months or more. Oregon also instituted an aldicarb-free sticker program.

Over the holiday, through active surveillance, officials received almost three hundred reports of people getting sick after eating watermelon in California, Washington, and Oregon. Sixty-one of these cases were confirmed aldicarb positive. One case was a physician who ate some watermelon and "just didn't feel right." The next day, he decided to have another go at it. This time, he felt dizzy and cloudy headed. Not one to learn from experience, or perhaps experimenting on himself, in the interest of science and public health, he tried again five hours later. This time he had diarrhea, nausea, vomiting, blurred vision, unsteadiness on his feet, and blurred thinking. His watermelon contained aldicarb at the lowest possible detection limit for the test used—0.01 parts per million.

Aldicarb is a highly toxic carbamate pesticide, licensed for use on cotton and some food crops, but not watermelon. This was not the first foodborne epidemic associated with aldicarb. In May 1985, hydroponically grown cucumbers in Canada were associated with two hundred reports and eighty-four probable cases of aldicarb poisoning. One possible explanation for the U.S. epidemic is that farmers used the pesticide illegally on watermelon. More likely, according to the investigators, is that aldicarb persisted in the soil from a previous season, when it had been applied to crops for which it is legally registered. Researchers have found aldicarb residues in potatoes, alfalfa, mint, mustard green, and radishes grown in soil that had been treated with aldicarb 450 days previously. Most of the soil samples were negative, even while the crops were positive, in an example of the phenomenon known as bioconcentration.

Heptachlor is a pesticide that was registered in the United States in 1952 and, after 1960, used against various agricultural pests and termites. After the standard laboratory animal testing suggested that heptachlor was carcinogenic, as well as toxic to the reproductive system and liver, the Food and Drug Administration (FDA) set a "zero" tolerance in foods. At the time, this meant an action level of 0.3 parts per million (ppm); although the test limits by 1982 were down below 0.05 ppm, and the World Health Organization recommended 0.15 ppm, the U.S. limits were still at 0.3—until, that is, the pineapple hit the fan.

When the Environmental Protection Agency banned all uses of heptachlor in 1976, some industries managed to beg, bully, or buy their way past the ban. Two of those exceptions that have later come back to haunt the regulators were for control of ants on pineapple plants and for use as a seed treatment.

On January 21, 1982, Albert Oda and his colleagues at the Hawaiian health department laboratory looked at the results of their routine milk testing. The milk samples were very high for heptachlor. Health department officials pondered this departure from normality and decided to keep their mouths shut. They sent the samples on to San Francisco for confirmation. When these results came back positive, they pondered again. They took more samples. These were also positive, leading them to believe that maybe they did not quite have enough samples yet.

Fifty-seven days after the initial positive results, the department, under pressure from an inquisitive newspaper, admitted that some milk was contaminated. Health officials recalled some milk and certified the rest as heptachlor free; when they tested the "free" milk, however, it also came up positive.

The story behind heptachlor use in pineapples is another lesson (do we really need more?) in ecology. Pineapple mealybugs (*Dysmicoccus brevipes*) damage pineapple plants. They have also developed a unique entomological society. The Hawaiian pineapple mealybugs reproduce through parthenogenesis (females produce female offspring without the help of males); ants harvest the honeydew that these mealybugs produce and provide a clean, safe (from parasites and predators) place for them to go about their happy, destructive lives. The pineapple companies used heptachlor not against the mealybugs directly but against their protectors, the ants. When Solomon admonished his readers to go learn from the ants, I suspect he was not thinking about these complex social relationships, certainly outside the bounds of what might be considered "traditional" family values.

In any case, while Dole and Del Monte were strategizing on how to get rid of the ants, agricultural researchers discovered how to mix chopped-up pineapple leaves with other things to make a nutritious cattle feed. This procedure appeared to be ecological efficiency at its best. Dole and Del Monte were supposed to wait a year after spraying before letting the dairymen on to the fields to harvest the leaves, but, well, things happen.

Anyway, said the health department director, who "retired" in the midst of the crisis, "emotionalism and hysteria" had clouded the public's ability to understand that the milk was safe. (To help promote public health, the governor replaced him with a former real-estate salesman). Short-term studies have not indicated any untoward effects in the Hawaiian population, but then no one is seriously worried about short-term effects anyway. Given that children drink far greater amounts of milk than adults and are more vulnerable because their bodies are growing, it is not at all clear, as the dean of the University of Hawaii's College of Tropical Agriculture said, that "continued consumption of milk with the reported heptachlor epoxide residue levels would not appear to constitute an unreasonable hazard." Potential damage to the dairy industry by bad publicity was, in his view, a much more serious concern.

The Hawaiian incident was not an isolated one. In 1984, the FDA in Mississippi notified the FDA office in New Orleans that a Mississippi firm was sending corn contaminated with aflatoxins (see chapter 12) to a company in New Orleans that made gasohol, a fuel-grade alcohol. How much aflatoxin goes into gasohol is of no concern to the FDA, but the New Orleans company would sell the mash left over from the process as animal feed, and there is an enforcement limit for aflatoxin levels in animal and human foods. The FDA monitored the process and discovered that the aflatoxin levels were too high for the mash to be allowed to slip into the food system.

In 1986, on one of their follow-up visits to review this alternative use of corn, FDA inspectors noticed some pink seeds mixed in with the other grain. The pink color indicated that the seeds had been treated with some chemical, perhaps a fungicide or other pesticide, and should not be eaten. Analyses of the grains showed levels of the pesticide heptachlor—in one sample a thousand times higher than the FDA's action level.

In March 1986, officials began testing milk from dairy farms that had bought feed from the New Orleans company. Dairy herds on nearly two hundred farms around Van Buren, Arkansas, were quarantined as a result of these tests. Nursing mothers were also tested and found to have measurable, though low, levels of heptachlor in their milk. The director of testing reassured them by saying that the lifetime additional risk of cancer for the nursing babies, beyond the one in twenty chance they already had just by living in the United States, was somewhere between one in a thousand and one in ten thousand. Members of farm families who had drunk the raw milk were found to have significantly higher heptachlor blood levels than other people in the area, but medical researchers could detect no immediate changes in their bodies.

Since Rachel Carson changed the public's outlook on the world of pesticides with her book *Silent Spring,* concerned citizens and scientists have mostly concerned themselves with the DDT type of organochlorine pesticides that persist and accumulate in the ecosystem. The main sources in the North American food supply have been animal fats. As a result of effective public pressure, the number of food items with DDT-like substances in them, and the levels at which they occur, have dropped dramatically, at least in the industrialized countries, since the late 1960s.

From a public health point of view, society is in a quandary. DDT is credited with saving millions of lives, both during World War II, when soldiers were sprayed, and in subsequent campaigns to eliminate malaria from large parts of the developing world. In early experiments, volunteers were even fed DDT powder, with no apparent ill effects. At the same time, the profligate and reckless use of DDT against just about any insect annoyance known to humanity resulted in widespread resistance to the drug in insect populations, compromising reproduction in a wide variety of birds, mammals, and insects, putting essential ecosystem services (such as pollination of wild and agricultural plants) at risk, and compromising the possibility of a sustainable human society on the planet.

Industrialized countries have replaced DDT with pesticides such as the organophosphates, which are less persistent, and so are less likely to show up in our food, but which are very toxic to the people that handle them. These people are often poor farm workers not protected by laws on child labor, minimum wage, workers' compensation, health, and the like. Thus, the risks of pesticide use have been shifted from urban consumers to farm workers and poor people in malaria-infested countries. Are the environmental concerns of wealthy urbanites simply a way of dumping on the poor of the world? I do not think they need to be, especially if we get away from the "economies of scale" solutions that industrialized countries have so obsessively pursued. Concerns about ecological health offer an opportunity to work with communities to develop socially just, biologically smarter, more sustainable, more targeted solutions.

Once food is safely off the farm and into stores and homes, consumers in many industrialized countries still want it to last at least a day or two. Few people want to shop for fresh produce every day. The solution to this problem: preservatives.

"No preservatives," says the label on my barbecue sauce. I look at the list of ingredients. Among other things, it includes vinegar (acetic acid), sugar, and salt—all preservatives—as well as some spices, which may also have antibacterial and hence preservative action. What is going on here? There is a legal definition of preservatives, geared to satisfy consumers and lawyers, and then there is the real world. What I guess the manufacturer of the sauce means is that it contains no recently synthesized chemicals.

In many developing countries, farmers may lose a third of their harvest to spoilage by pests and bacteria. In industrialized countries, the canning jars for tomatoes and vegetables, which demand a higher commitment to housework and hence less commitment to the institutions that want our bodies to maximize their profits, are no longer culturally acceptable. The cool cellar for potatoes and carrots is neither feasible nor esthetically consonant with apartment life. People want their food to look absolutely fresh and not to spoil the day they buy it and also to have the illusion of no preservatives. Not asking for much, eh?

Meat processors add nitrites to ham to keep the meat pink, to add flavor, to prevent the fat from going rancid, and, most important, to prevent *Clostridium botulinum,* the organism that causes botulism, from multiplying. Nitrites also combine with other food ingredients to form substances called nitrosamines, which cause cancer in a wide variety of species. To complicate matters, nitrates, a related group of compounds that our bodies can make into nitrites, are found at very high levels (more than ten times that of ham) in beets and lettuce.

Do consumers want fresh salads at a salad bar in the middle of winter? Hey, that's easy. If you add sulfites to freshly cut vegetables, you can prevent what is called enzymatic browning. You will also destroy some thiamine in the food and give hundreds of people across North America, primarily asthmatics, an allergic reaction. But heck, there are puffers for asthma, and as for the thiamine, why did God invent vitamin supplements anyway?

Consumers want sweet food but do not want cavities or calories. So the food scientists produced cyclamates—until the 1970s, when tumors in rats caused cyclamates to be banned—and saccharin, which may or may not cause cancer. After that came aspartame, which was approved by the commissioner of the Food and Drug Administration of the United States against the advice of his scientific advisory panel. Four months after he had approved it, the commissioner was working for the advertising agency that handled the aspartame account. Side effects of the sweetener reported by consumers since it hit the market are mostly neurological, ranging from headaches to mood changes to seizures. Ironically, there is some evidence now that people who use artificial sweeteners may actually gain weight. Their bodies crave carbohydrates, so they eat something artificially sweetened. While the taste buds can be fooled, the brain is not so easily misled and demands more, the real stuff this time. Our brains need sugar to function properly. Hence people eat more and gain weight.

Antibacterial drugs, pesticides, and preservatives have helped humanity produce food and alleviate suffering in animals and people worldwide. These chemicals have made major contributions to the control of disease and increases in food production. One could argue that less disease and more food have contributed to the population explosion and hence the current environmental crisis, but I think that argument is, at the very least, ethically suspect.

Humanity has been given the power to save lives and alter how food is produced and in so doing is faced with many serious moral questions about prolonging life versus quality of life, sexual behavior, abortion, population control, food production, and environmental and social degradation. Almost every case of foodborne disease is a natural consequence of interdependence, a matter of what goes around comes around. The questions raised are difficult, and there are no easy answers.

If food safety issues are taken seriously, they are at heart ecological, social, political, and economic questions. If we as a human species want to resolve these issues, we must walk the fine lines between cure and coffin, knowing that there are no perfect answers, only imperfect people. Otherwise it is just a game.

11

DANCING CAT
MEETS
CADMIUM
CARROT

HEAVY METALS

O N DECEMBER 4, 1969, an eight-year-old girl from Alamogordo, New Mexico, began suffering from incoordination, vision problems, and a gradual decrease in consciousness, until she lapsed into a coma. Within a month, her thirteen-year-old brother and her older sister followed her to the hospital with similar symptoms. An investigation showed that in September their father had fed some mercury-treated grain to his eighteen pigs, twelve of which died and two of which stayed blind. The other four looked okay, so he butchered one of them and, during that autumn, served it up to the family.

Organic mercury compounds (the most toxic form of the metal) were used after 1914 and into the 1960s as a treatment to prevent fungal infections in cereal grains to be used as seeds.

As you might imagine, poor farmers could not always keep the seeds for planting and sometimes ate them directly or fed them to livestock, which was then eaten. As the result of such practices, epidemics of mercury poisoning occurred in the United States, Guatemala, Pakistan, and Iraq (where according to one report, 6,500 people were affected in 1971–72, with over four hundred deaths).

Swedish researchers plotted the concentration of mercury in the feathers of terrestrial birds from 1840 through the 1970s. Levels remained low and constant until about 1946, when mercury seed treatments began to be used. After that, levels of mercury in these birds rapidly increased. After 1965, when this method of treating seeds was stopped, the levels in the seed-eating birds began to decrease. In fish-eating birds, however, levels have gradually increased since the beginning of the industrial revolution, which should not be a surprise to anyone who knows about the travels of mercury in aquatic systems.

Today the major source of methyl (organic) mercury in the diet of most people around the world is from fish, particularly big fish at the top of the food chain, such as shark and swordfish. In people, the metal is almost completely absorbed from the gut and crosses both the placenta to the fetus and the blood-brain barrier, which is supposed to protect your brain. It takes seventy to eighty days for half the mercury in your body to be cleared.

The biggest and most tragic epidemic of mercury poisoning occurred in Japan after World War II. In the late 1950s, Minamata disease emerged in communities near Minamata, in southwestern Japan. The ways in which this disease presented itself had all the hallmarks of a horror movie. Dead fish were found floating in Minamata Bay. Octopus and cuttlefish were so weakened that children could catch them by hand. Seagulls and crows dropped into the water. Cats would stagger about as if drunk, whirl suddenly, and dash away in a zigzag manner, or simply collapse. Locals referred to this as dancing-cat disease.

In people, numbness in the limbs and around the mouth was followed by difficulty with hand movements, such as using chopsticks, and general incoordination. Victims went on to develop slurred speech, disturbances of vision and hearing, difficulty swallowing, paralysis, convulsions, and death. A large number of infants with cerebral-palsy-like syndromes were born in the affected area.

By 1959, investigators knew that all these manifestations came from eating mercury-contaminated fish and that the Chiso Corporation was dumping mercury into Minamata Bay. The inhabitants were told to quit eating fish. The pollution continued. By 1962, people thought the emergency was taken care of, and they resumed their normal diet. Investigators were still uncovering cases in the mid- to late 1970s. Based on their evidence, they wondered if one could talk about "safe" or "acceptable" levels.

There are some metals, such as iron, zinc, copper, and selenium, which we need in trace amounts. It's the ones we don't need—especially heavy metals like lead, mercury, and cadmium (to which I might add the likes of Iron Butterfly and Led Zeppelin)—that pose a hazard to us.

During the postwar years, in Japan, several hundred women who worked in, and ate from, certain rice fields, developed a severe, very painful, and often fatal disease of the bones referred to by those affected as *itai-itai* (ouch-ouch) disease. The rice fields in question were irrigated with cadmium-contaminated water from a zinc mine. Cadmium attacks the kidneys. Although only about 5 percent of cadmium is absorbed by people, it takes about thirty years for half the cadmium to be cleared from your body once it's there. Cadmium occurs naturally throughout the world and has always posed a health risk to people who lived in certain areas or worked with metals, but we human beings seem to have made a special effort to redistribute the risks and bring cadmium (like lead and mercury) into our own special social systems and ecosystems. We concentrate cadmium through industrial processes, in batteries and electroplating, and as a contaminant in other metals we use. We also sometimes effectively recycle it by using contaminated sewage sludge to grow our crops. Having invited some of these poisons to live with us, we are going to have to deal with them in our recycling programs.

Smoking remains a major source of cadmium exposure, but for those of us to whom inhaling burning tobacco leaves is as pleasurable as breathing car exhaust or a traveling companion's flatulence, our major source of exposure is through cereals and vegetables, especially root vegetables. In Canada, horse livers seem to have very high levels, and Agriculture and Agri-Food Canada has disallowed horse offal as human food. This is not a purely Canadian phenomenon; an investigation in China found that cadmium residues in horses were fifteen to seventy times as high as in cattle, swine, or sheep, and similar phenomena have been noted in the United States.

Global trade has introduced some new twists into an old story. Lisa Deutsch and her colleagues in Stockholm recently reported that cadmium was increasing in Swedish soils because animal feeds were being imported from ecosystems in other parts of the world (eastern Europe, Brazil, Southeast Asia) where the metal was more common. These feeds were being imported in part to maintain the traditional agricultural landscape of the Swedish countryside and because the feed inputs such as soybeans could not be grown in Sweden. Thus, not only were uncritical policies to promote sustainable agriculture in Sweden offloading environmental costs (such as land clearing and crop intensification in Brazil), but they were also having negative effects in the very areas they were designed to protect.

One can get a dose of lead from various sources, including, at least until recently, leaded paints and gas. Still, about 60 percent of lead intake in the United States is probably through food. The use of lead solder in canned foods has stopped in most industrialized countries, but some ceramic glazes continue to be a problem.

Aluminum is found in higher levels in the brains of people who have died of Alzheimer's disease, but nobody has been able to show convincingly that it causes Alzheimer's. Indeed, if there is a connection it is an indirect one; in the occupational health literature, exposure to pesticides, but not to aluminium, has been associated with the disease. Still, I was enough persuaded to buy a stainless steel pot for cooking my tomatoes, cabbage, and applesauce (which soak it up more than other foods), but not enough to get rid of my aluminum pots. Maybe that is a sign that I already have brain damage. In any case, buffered aspirin (which I can live without), baking powder (give up my waffles and muffins? actually, I did, but in response to an egg allergy, not because of concerns about aluminum) and tea (which I am not about to forgo) are far greater sources of aluminum in our diets than cooking pots.

Pentachlorophenol (PCP) comes from a family of chemicals used as wood preservatives because they can kill so many life-forms (bacteria, insects, fungi, plants). Although PCP is poisonous to people in high doses, some low-level effects that people have associated with it are probably the result of contamination with dioxins. The worst effect of the PCP itself is probably a musty odor. When it does enter the food chain, it is from animals raised on treated wood shavings or in treated-wood buildings.

Polychlorinated dibenzodioxins (PCDDs) and polychlorinated dibenzofurans (PCDFs), sometimes called dioxins, are really an extended family of more than two hundred compounds with no commercial uses. These have entered the environment and hence the food chain from incineration plants, high-temperature industrial processes, the pulp-and-paper industry, and traffic exhausts. Seventeen of these compounds are reported to be toxic. In animal tests, they cause cancers and affect the reproductive

and immune systems. Acute effects in people seen after industrial accidents (such as the explosion of a factory in Seveso, Italy)
and contamination of food sources (such as rice oil in Yusho,
Japan) include chloracne, measurable disturbances in peripheral
nerve function, fatigue, and liver toxicity. As with most manufactured chemicals in the food chain, the chronic effects have
been much more difficult to demonstrate. Although we seem to
accumulate dioxins in our bodies more efficiently than rabbits
and rats, there is no strong evidence that they are as toxic to
us as to those species. Most human exposure to dioxin (80 to
100 percent) comes through food, mostly fish, and some through
meat and milk.

Hexachlorobenzene (HCB) is one of twelve chlorinated ben-
zenes that have been used throughout the world for a wide
variety of pesticidal applications. One hundred and thirty-five
pesticides and more than twenty industrial chemicals are suspected of being able to form HCB as a contaminant. HCB is also
present in commercial-grade PCP and has a longer half-life in
dairy cows (about fifty days) than PCP itself (a few days). HCB
was introduced in 1945 as a fungicide for use on seeds and in
soil. In the late 1950s and early 1960s, poor farmers in Turkey ate
HCB-treated seed grains, resulting in an epidemic of a disease
syndrome that included sensitivity reactions to sunlight and
effects on the nervous system. A high incidence of stillbirths
and high infant mortality was observed in women exposed during gestation and lactation. The health effects were severe, but
no cancer occurred, illustrating at the very least the limitations
of using cancer as our only measure of concern.

Because of the known effects of HCB at high doses in people,
and low doses in animals, together with its persistence in the
environment and its tendency to bioaccumulate (up to ten thousand times in some aquatic systems), it is no longer produced
or used as a fungicide in most parts of the world. Still, a lot
of it enters the system as a waste by-product in the production

of some pesticides and chlorinated solvents. Again, our main dietary sources of HCB are fish, meat, and milk.

Two widely used industrial compounds, polychlorinated biphenyls (PCBs) and polybrominated biphenyls (PBBs), have caused several major foodborne outbreaks during the 1970s. Both PCBs and PBBs undergo biomagnification.

PCBs were used extensively throughout the industrialized world, mainly by the electrical industry and in coolant systems, for about fifty years; the public was assured by people who should have known better that these were "closed systems." There are no closed systems on this planet, or in this universe, as far as I can tell. These chemicals became ubiquitous in the environment. PCBs were first synthesized in 1881 but were only commercially exploited, with a vengeance it seems, after 1930. In their heyday, they were used in plastics, paints, heat exchangers, kiss-proof lipsticks, and carbonless copy papers. Until the mid-1960s, when researchers began to find PCBs in fish and wild birds, it was assumed that these chemicals appeared only in these supposedly controlled closed systems.

In 1968, in Japan, rice oil that had been added to poultry feed was found to be responsible for the deaths of 400,000 chickens. It turned out that the rice oil contained PCBs and, to complicate matters, dioxins. An "objective" scientist might ask: given that it is bad for chickens, is it bad for people? After the epidemic in chickens, medical epidemiologists determined that the same brand of rice oil was causing chronic and sometimes debilitating effects in people: chloracne, nausea, vomiting, peripheral numbness, and disorders of the nervous system and the gut. As a result of incidents such as this one and the Michigan PBB incident (described below), much tighter controls were put on industrial chemicals; and PCBs were banned.

In Canada and the United States, freshwater fish are reported to be the major accumulators of PCBs. Although they are no longer manufactured or sold in the United States, PCBs continue to enter the food chain from various contaminated environmental sources, such as sediments in some streams. Environmental contamination persists from accidental spills and leakage from electrical transformers and capacitors, disposal of contaminated sewage, and wrapping and packaging material made of recycled paper that contains PCBs. Studies from around the world show that the body burden (the amount stored in fats in people) has been decreasing over the past two decades. The regulations are having an effect. Still, it will be many years yet before we know the whole story on these chemicals.

In the summer of 1973, in Michigan, five hundred to a thousand pounds of Firemaster, the brand name for polybrominated biphenyls (a fire retardant), were accidentally added to some animal feed instead of Nutrimaster, a feed additive. Effects on animals throughout Michigan were insidious and widespread, and it took at least eight months to determine their cause. Fortunately, one of the farmers who was most seriously affected had a degree in chemical engineering and had once worked for a chemical company.

Even after the culprit was identified as PBB, it took another year and a half to find all the affected farms and quarantine them. The government was unsure what levels in food to consider "acceptable," and hence when to invoke regulatory action, because no one had had any experience with PBBs as toxins in food. Authorities also lacked good testing procedures and toxicological experiments. During this time, thousands of people were exposed to contaminated milk, meat, and eggs. A wide range of human symptoms was reported, including numbness, balance problems, nausea, stomach problems, changes in appetite, irritability, and headaches. No one seems to have discovered what the full range of PBB-induced problems is. Some reports have concluded that there are, in fact, no effects.

PBBs are like many of the chemicals in the human food chain: people kind of grew up with them, and they are all around us, so it is hard to tell what their effects are and how much of what we think they are doing is simply a normal side effect of being human. Am I irritable because I had a hard day at work or am belatedly going through a midlife crisis, or is it the PBBs, the dioxins, or the cadmium?

The massive increase in the production of new chemicals, with which no species has had any evolutionary experience, has created as many problems as it has solutions to problems. How can one eat intelligently in this kind of world, where these industrial chemicals are floating around? Is there no safe place? We shall all die, one way or another, and that should give us some pause before we panic and embrace either eating only pure California-grown air-sprouts (with *Salmonella* or *E. coli* dressing) or giving industries their amoral way. Better testing procedures, regulations, risk assessments, and mathematical modes can offer some guidance, but a better understanding of ecology in general should give us some pause.

The message, again and again, from changing patterns of foodborne diseases, is that questions we need to ask as a society are more fundamental than can simply be answered through a series of technical procedures and regulations. More than many human activities, the patterns of intoxicants in our food should cause us to look carefully at our entire economy. Heavy metals in our foods are the result of activities that would appear to have little to do with food production itself but rather with the context in which that production and distribution take place. We need to develop just, open, multi-ocular ways of thinking and acting. And we need to ask what kind of a world we want to live in.

12

BREADWICHES, PEANUT LIVERS, AND CANCER-FREE AIRLINE SNACKS

MYCOTOXINS

A PEANUT BUTTER on rye sandwich may seem to be a health food made in heaven, or at least in California, but consider the demons that lurk even here.

The description of ergotism, a disease produced by fungal toxins (called mycotoxins) in rye bread, could just as easily be a description by some hellfire preacher of the torments of a soul damned to Hades. A holy fire consumes the sufferer, and so the victim feels an intense internal heat and thirst; the skin breaks out in ulcers, the limbs feel as if they are burning, and it feels as though ants and mice are crawling under the skin. Finally, the hands, arms, legs, and feet turn black, and blindness and (understandable under the circumstances) dementia set in.

The description of this illness goes back to the Greeks in 430 BC, but reaches its most intense metaphysical dimensions in the European Middle Ages. To seek healing from their fire, people left their homes (and their local rye bread) to visit the shrine of the hermit St. Anthony, renowned for his healing powers in Dauphine, France; St. Anthony's remains had been transferred there in 1070. The sufferers were indeed healed, though it took some six hundred years before they figured out that the culprits were the ergot alkaloids produced by the mold *Claviceps purpurea* in the rye bread. It was almost two hundred years after the Salem, Massachusetts witch trials that Linda Caporael could ask, in the title of an article in the respected journal *Science*, "Ergotism: the Satan loosed in Salem?" There is something at once silly and frightening in the idea of the devil as a loaf of contaminated rye bread, the kind of idea that might be dreamed up by the medieval mystic Meister Eckhart in collaboration with Monty Python. Such is the strange, terrible, and wonderful nature of the world we live in.

The last epidemic attributed to ergot in Europe occurred in France, in 1951, when two hundred people became ill after consuming bread made from contaminated rye flour. Twenty-five people suffered delirium, and four people died.

Once the black or purple masses (ergots) were recognized as the source of the poison, such infested grains could be, and usually were, avoided. Rapid harvesting and drying of grains, and the use of fungicides make this a rare disease today. Those cases of ergot poisoning that do occur now are more likely related to its medicinal uses. One derivative of the ergot alkaloids is the treatment of choice for migraine headaches; my wife says her headaches went away, but she felt as if her body was floating above the bed. This effect is a reminder that another compound, the 1960s hallucinogen LSD, belongs to the same family. As a rural veterinarian, I used another relative to inject into cows postcalving, to encourage (rather forcefully) the uterus to contract: in this and many other ways, modern medicine has tamed and channeled the devils of earlier eras.

Fungi are all around us, producing spores that cause us to sneeze and wheeze and that decorate our leftovers with carpets of green and black in the refrigerator. As you might imagine, they have many opportunities to participate in our environmental marriages. If some species, like *Claviceps*, attack foods in the field, others wait until we have harvested the food and placed it into storage. The fungi that produce aflatoxins, *Aspergillus* species, are of this type.

On a recent flight across the Pacific, between the three mediocre movies, braced with a gin and tonic, I examined the little snack pack I had been given. "No aflatoxin," said the label. "High Vitamin A. Low fat." Labels can tell a person a lot about what societies value, or at least what some people think that other people think is important. The high vitamin A and low fat I could understand. But no aflatoxin? Who cared? Would any of my fellow passengers even know what aflatoxins were?

Aflatoxin poisoning no doubt occurred as a sporadic problem in farm animals long before it was recognized as such. Then, in 1960–61, a strange affliction, called, in a spasm of scientific imagination, turkey-X disease, seemed to spread through the young turkey poultry population of south England. Millions of poults, as well as chicks and ducklings, died. The cause was eventually traced to peanut meal (sometimes called by the less informative name Rossetti meal, after the boat that brought the meal from Brazil). Since that time, aflatoxins have become the most thoroughly studied of the thousands of toxins that various molds produce, and the ones most likely to make headlines.

Aflatoxins are thought to play a role in suppressing immune systems in children in southern Africa who eat mold-infested grains. This immune suppression interferes with childhood vaccination programs against diseases like polio, measles, diphtheria, and mumps. The mycotoxin-induced immune suppression also makes them more likely to get sick from malaria. In Thailand, aflatoxins were implicated in Reye's syndrome, a rare but invariably fatal disease of young children, who go into a coma and convulsions. In North America, Reye's syndrome has been described as a sequela of influenza in some children who take aspirin, which led to a massive switch to acetaminophen by parents of young children. Acetaminophen causes kidney damage, but I guess a small probability of a coma is worse than a small probability of impaired kidneys.

Although North American public health workers tend to worry about chronic exposures to aflatoxins, massive, acutely toxic, one-time exposures are greater concerns in some developing countires. In the mid-1970s, people in more than two hundred villages in India were afflicted with vomiting, abdominal pain, and wrecked livers; more than a hundred people died. In Kenya, in 2004, more than three hundred people suffered acute liver disease, and 125 of them died, from eating maize (as corn is called in most of the world outside of Canada, the United States, and Australia) infested with aflatoxins. Maize was imported into Africa from South America, where traditions for growing and storing maize are ancient. In Africa, maize is often eaten as a mash, on a daily basis, as a food staple, the way North American eat potatoes. Some might wonder if the aflatoxin problems in Africa are a result of this crop transfer into cultures that do not have long traditions of working with it. In both culture and ecology, context is everything. North American regulators have developed stringent screening procedures for aflatoxins (recall the story of how they found heptachlor in Arkansas corn, while looking for aflatoxins); as well, we usually eat our corn in highly processed forms, in which the mycotoxins are at least partially destroyed.

Aflatoxins have sparked intense concern in North America because, even at very low levels, there is good evidence that, along with hepatitis B virus and some other factors, they cause liver cancer. Some of the evidence for this relationship is epidemiological. In those parts of the world where aflatoxin contamination of food is high, there are also high levels of liver cancer. There is also toxicological evidence. Rats fed aflatoxins develop cancer. That aflatoxins have chosen that good old American food, peanut butter, as the vehicle for visiting our bodies, has raised a few hackles. Dr. Strangelove might suggest a fundamentalist (Muslim, Hindu, atheist, or Christian—pick your poison) plot. If it were a man-made chemical, we would certainly see consumer protests about it.

In a sense, aflatoxins are man-made chemicals. Fungal toxins develop in our foods because of how we grow and store them; warm, moist conditions are best. Aflatoxins happen to prefer nuts and seeds. When people harvest nuts and seeds, store them for a long time, and ship them all over the world, they are creating an aflatoxin production system. Urban consumers and their food industry allies do not live next door to the poor peanut farmers who grow the peanuts and are not about to pay more money for better drying and storage facilities. It is a gentle, though sometimes deadly, reminder that, vegetarian or not, we live in a global food distribution society where the natural consequence of not caring about our neighbors is that we get sick.

Studies in the United States in the 1970s and 1980s found that three-quarters of all peanut butter samples tested had some aflatoxins, and about 10 percent had levels high enough to kick the regulators into gear. Roasting will destroy about 50 percent of aflatoxins in food, and large commercial companies have developed procedures to process nuts and to test the products so as to meet stiff new regulatory standards. Sadly, small organic processors do not always have access to, or cannot afford, appropriate technologies. Again, there are trade-offs between safety related to mycotoxins, the possibility of widespread bacterial contamination of industrial products (as has occurred), the health benefits of eating nuts, the increased nut allergies that emerge in populations that eat a lot of nuts, and the ecological and social benefits of small-scale organic agriculture.

In the 1990s, fumonisins, mycotoxins produced by the *Fusarium* species, were found to contaminate corn and maize all over the world. Fumonisins cause kidney and liver damage in pretty well all the species in which they have been tested. They are known to cause pulmonary edema (water in the lungs) in pigs, and leucoencephalomalacia (basically turning the brain into mush) in horses. There are reports from South Africa, where maize is often a staple food, eaten on a daily basis without any industrial processing, that these toxins cause cancer of the esophagus in people.

One other mycotoxin-related disease is primarily of historical interest, but it is still instructive. In the former Soviet Union in the years just after 1913, and again, with a vengeance, in 1941 to 1945, epidemics of a disease called alimentary toxic aleukia (ATA) spread from Siberia to Europe. The sickness would begin in May, build to a peak in June, and then trail off through the summer. Within a few hours after eating bread, the affected person would have a peppery taste and burning sensation in the mouth and throat. Within days, nausea, vomiting, and diarrhea followed, and then, as the bone marrow degenerated over weeks and months, the person would develop hemorrhages and ulcers, and the flesh would start rotting.

This horrible disease is attributed to toxins from mold growing in crops that were left in the fields over the winter and harvested only after spring thaw. The stories my mother told me of the crops left in the fields as war stormed through their villages in Russia somehow give this disease a particular edge for me. And when I hear of war once again tearing the fabric of the former communist states, or the devastation wreaked by post-9/11 battles fought in Third World countries, I fear that one day soon I will open some staid medical journal and read about an "interesting outbreak" of ATA.

Fungi and the toxins they produce prefer warm, wet environments, although, as a quick perusal of the wasteland in our refrigerator will show, the warm part is not essential. Most foods will support fungal growth and mycotoxin production, but damaged or stressed plants, as one might find after a drought, particularly various nuts, corn, and figs, are more hospitable to fungi than foods from animals.

Finally, there are a few unexpected substances that inhibit these death-dealing fungi: cinnamon, cloves, and mustard, at normal levels; thyme, garlic, oregano, allspice, and anise at high levels; and foods that contain a fair amount of acid or that have had acid added. I am thinking of starting a mycotoxin-free-food franchise in Toronto. I could serve spaghetti with tomato sauce and lots of garlic, followed by pumpkin pie, perhaps, with just a little mustard added. I could also set out bowls of those aflatoxin-free sesame snacks I got on the plane from Japan as appetizers.

Oh, and another good way to stop some of the more serious mycotoxicoses: stop war.

13

THERE
IS A
CRACK IN
EVERYTHING

RADIOACTIVE
CONTAMINANTS

S OF THE time I am writing this, the world has not seen any major nuclear reactor accidents such as the one at Chernobyl in 1986. Many people seem to have forgotten that accident, and the nuclear industry is again parading itself as a world savior. At one time, nuclear energy was good because, well, it was nuclear, and that sounded cool. Now, nuclear power is paraded as the "green" alternative, keeping the global greenhouse cool and the energy-hungry global economy hot. North Koreans and Iranians are not the only gals skipping through the woods with their big baskets. I confess that I am skeptical about all these green and happy future scenarios. Nuclear power plants are awfully big baskets with a lot of eggs in them. There is a wolf in the woods on the way to Grandma's house. Will the basket get dropped, on purpose or accidentally? Of course.

Douglas Adams, author of *Hitchhiker's Guide to the Galaxy*, once said that the main difference between things that can go wrong and those that can't possibly go wrong is that when the "can't possibly go wrong" ones go wrong, they are unfixable. This is a useful thought to pair with singer-songwriter Leonard Cohen's phrase that "there is a crack in everything." I think it's worth reviewing what we might be faced with in case there is, heaven help us, another impossible accident.

The probability that our food will become contaminated with radionuclides from a nuclear disaster may be small (though with the collapse of the Soviet empire and the proliferation of reactionary nationalism, that probability may have increased). Nevertheless, the effects can be serious throughout the world, and are worth giving at least passing consideration.

Various kinds of nuclear disasters can occur. Nuclear bombs may be tested—not, of course, in Paris or Washington, but in the South Pacific islands. Or we may drop nuclear weapons as acts of war. Since cures for the effects of radiation are based largely on wishful thinking, prevention is not only possible but, from a medical viewpoint, essential.

Nuclear bombs may also be dropped accidentally. Such nuclear accidents are sometimes referred to as "broken arrows." If I were a suspicious person, I would wonder, why arrows? Why not broken M-16s? In any case, between 1950 and 1980, the United States officially reported twenty-two broken arrows over various parts of the continental United States, the Pacific and Atlantic oceans, Greenland, and Spain. Many of the lost weapons were never recovered. A 1968 crash in North Star Bay, Greenland, scattered plutonium over a wide area, and Danish clean-up workers were exposed to it. The former Soviet Union no doubt also lost many nuclear weapons, but these losses have not been publicly documented. It is perhaps appropriate to thank

God, or at least the laws of probability, that no major explosions or inadvertent wars have resulted from these accidents.

Finally, accidents may occur in nuclear power or weapons plants, in storage sites, or during the transport of materials. Several major accidents of this type, and many minor ones, have occurred over the last thirty years, including those at Chelyabinsk, USSR, in 1957–58, Windscale (now Sellafield), England, in 1957, Idaho Falls and Three Mile Island, USA, in 1961 and 1979, respectively, and Chernobyl, USSR, in 1986.

What we know about radionuclides in the food chain has been accumulated from follow-ups to the accidents I mention above, as well as from experimental studies, from field surveys done around uranium mines and nuclear power plants, and from food surveys carried out in the 1950s and 1960s in response to concerns about fallout from atmospheric testing of nuclear weapons. Results of these surveys have provided much useful information about naturally occurring radionuclides in the earth's crust. Some of these, such as the uranium, thorium, and actinium series, each of which end in a different stable isotope of lead, have been present since the time the earth was formed. Others, such as carbon-14 and beryllium-10, are formed continuously by reactions between cosmic and solar radiation and stable nuclei. Some human populations, in parts of France, India, and Brazil, and in the northern circumpolar region, have historically been subject to higher levels of natural radiation than others. These natural radionuclides, present heterogeneously in the earth's crust, have since been joined by radionuclides produced during atmospheric weapons testing, resulting in what is called background radiation.

Many measures of radioactivity are reported in the literature, and it is easy to get lost among the trees and not see the shape of the forest. Because all the international regulations are stated in standard international and metric units, I am going to stick to those here, and if you, as a reader, find that this gets too technical, then skim over the details. In this case, the devil is not so much in the details as in the big picture, and the big picture is this: more than two decades after a single nuclear-plant accident, scientists continue to find widespread contamination in the environment (that is, food).

The becquerel, the gray, and the sievert may sound like seafoods but are in fact useful measures. The becquerel measures the strength of the radioactive source, specifically, the number of radioactive disintegrations per unit time. One becquerel (Bq) = one disintegration/second. The dose—more correctly, the absorbed dose, defined as how much energy per unit mass is deposited in a material—is measured in grays. One gray (Gy) = one joule/kg. Finally, the dose equivalent gives an indication of the biological effects of an absorbed dose of radiation in tissue. Measured in sieverts (Sv), the dose equivalent is a function of the dose in grays times the quality factor (QF), which measures the ability of a given dose to cause biological damage. The quality factor is not an exact adjustment but provides an approximate basis of comparison of the same absorbed dose from different sources.

We can use these measures to assess three important questions. How much radioactivity is there in the food (Bq/kg)? How much of that radioactivity, if ingested, will be absorbed (Gy)? If given a choice between two radioactive foods, which one should we eat or feed to our animals? (The one with the lower Sv level.) Clearly the absorbed dose measurements, inexact as they may be, are the most important for making practical decisions in the face of a disaster.

The International Commission on Radiological Protection (ICRP) has suggested that dose equivalents, excluding natural background and medically related radiation, should not exceed 5 millisieverts (mSv) in a given year, 1 mSv per year on average, and 70 mSv over a lifetime. Many countries have created action levels based on these guidelines, but it should be borne in mind that average levels are created for average populations, which

may not exist. As with World Health Organization residue recommendations, we should view these as working guidelines, not
to be used slavishly and without common sense.

Before we jump into the meat of this matter, we should clear
up two other definitions. The physical half-life indicates how
long it takes for half a quantity of radioactive material to decay
into another substance; the product may or may not be radioactive. The biological half-life is an estimate of how long it takes
for a given biological system, usually an individual animal or
plant, to rid itself of half the initial radioactive material. The
physical half-life is therefore a characteristic of the substance
itself, while the biological half-life is a function of how the substance is metabolized in the body.

In addition, the ecological half-life, or effective half-life, is
an estimate of how long a given radionuclide will persist in an
ecosystem or food chain. For instance, the physical half-life
of cesium-137 is about thirty years. The biological half-life of
cesium-137 in the muscles of individual reindeer is only about
two weeks, and the ecological half-life in the reindeer-lichen
ecosystem is about ten to fifteen years, reflecting the long biological half-life in lichen. Thus, for short-term management of
farm animals, the biological half-life is very important, while
for the long-term assurance of a safe food supply, the ecological
half-life, often closely approximated by physical half-life, should
take precedence. Iodine-131, however, has a physical half-life of
only eight days but has a biological half-life in humans of two to
four months, and so preventing exposure is critical.

Finally, when thinking about chemicals in ecosystems, we
need to keep in mind the reality of bioaccumulation and biomagnification—the accumulation of substances in animals and
plants and their increased concentration as they move up the
predator-prey food pyramid (see earlier discussions of cigua-
toxia and DDT for more on this). Radionuclides may accumulate
in certain parts of the food chains.

A great many radionuclides, or radioactive isotopes, may be produced in nuclear accidents. After Chernobyl, iodine-131, cesium-134, cesium-137, and small amounts of ruthenium-103, tellurium-132, and strontium-90 were detected in several European countries. Strontium-90 has traditionally been associated with fallout from weapons testing.

In all cases, retention of radionuclides in biological systems depends on the amount of stable, nonradioactive isotope present and the metabolic interactions between the radionuclide and the stable form. One of the rationales for treatment of animals or people who have been exposed to radionuclides is to provide stable isotopes to compete for uptake with the radionuclide. Biologically, iodine-131 is rapidly absorbed, follows the body's iodine pathways, and concentrates in the thyroid. In people, most iodine-131 is excreted via urine. Cesium mimics potassium and is distributed throughout muscle tissue; if offered both potassium and cesium, the body preferentially retains cesium. Strontium is metabolized similarly to calcium, being incorporated into bony tissue, and thus has a slow turnover time in the body. Ruthenium-103 and tellurium-132 are poorly absorbed and thus pose the least risk.

If we focus on reactor-related accidents, with Chernobyl as our case type, then the activities of iodine-131 and cesium-137 may be considered useful indicators of the shape of the disaster and the kind of responses called for.

Aerial distribution of radionuclides depends on the quantity of radioactive material released, how high the material is thrown into the atmosphere, and wind and weather patterns, which affect how widely it is dispersed. The actual terrestrial distribution of the fallout is then in large measure determined by precipitation patterns, which in turn may be affected by smoke, other particulate matter in the air, and topography. Because of these variables, radioactive hot spots are unevenly distributed. A "tree umbrella" effect was seen after Chernobyl, in which a heavy tree cover captured the rain, and the radioactivity, before it reached the ground.

Once the radionuclides are on the ground, the organic and mineral content of the soil influences their distribution and passage into the food chain. Plants grown on soils with high organic matter and low clay content, for instance, are expected to experience high uptake of radiocesium for many years. Clay soils tend to have a higher cesium-binding capacity and therefore do not recycle it into plants as quickly.

Plant uptake of radionuclides depends on the radionuclide involved, the stage of plant growth, the type of plant, and the soil conditions. After Chernobyl, broad, leafy plants such as spinach contained high levels of iodine-131 in Belgium; 10 to 40 percent of radioactive iodine deposited on plant leaves may be directly absorbed. In contrast, very low levels of radiocesium were found on spinach in Sweden, reflecting not only the radionuclide type but also differences in stage of growth and soil type. Lichens and some mushrooms depend on surface, rather than soil, moisture, making them particularly vulnerable to contaminated rainfall. Furthermore, lichens grow very slowly and thus may gather and concentrate radionuclides over a long period of time. The effective ecological half-life of radiocesium in some parts of the Canadian Arctic has been estimated at ten to twelve years. Root uptake of cesium-137 is lower than leaf uptake, so cereals grown on soil that was tilled after the Chernobyl accident but before planting generally had low levels of contamination.

The uptake of radionuclides by various animals again depends on a whole complex of interactions, but the type of feed they eat is a major determinant. Because they eat lichens, reindeer and caribou are particularly vulnerable; in Norway and Sweden, levels of contamination jumped from 200 to 300 Bq/kg before Chernobyl to, in a few cases, over 60,000 Bq/kg after the accident.

Sheep and goats eat closer to the ground than cattle or horses, and goats browse, so the small ruminants are the most vulnerable farm animals. The biological half-life of radiocesium in cattle is about five weeks and in sheep about two weeks, but some sheep in the United Kingdom were still registering levels of greater than 1,000 Bq/kg when they came down from highland pastures in April 2006. In Norway, sheep were still registering 7,000 Bq/kg in October 2006. These elevated rates must reflect, then, persistent environmental exposure. The Norwegians think the high levels in 2006 were the result of a wet year and lots of mushrooms, which tend to take up radioactivity.

Commercial pigs and poultry tend to be fed prepared or imported feed, and to be kept indoors, and are therefore more protected. Dairy cattle kept indoors and fed stored feeds are less likely to be contaminated than those at pasture.

After Chernobyl, milk from sheep and goats was more heavily contaminated than cows' milk, posing special problems for control, because milk from small ruminants tends to be distributed outside the normally regulated channels. When milk is separated, radionuclides concentrate more in the whey than in the curd. In cheese, over a three-month period iodine-131 tends to disappear, and cesium-137 (and strontium-90, if present) tends to concentrate, a function largely of their different physical half-lives and the fluid weight loss in the cheese over time.

Finally, radionuclide contamination of fish depends on the water type and quality and the feeding habits and growth rates of the fish. In Sweden, freshwater fish were more heavily contaminated than marine fish after Chernobyl, partly because of the dilution effect of the ocean but also because of the concentration of potassium in seawater, which is about a hundred times that of fresh water. Fish with slow growth rates in northern, nutrient-poor lakes were the most vulnerable. Both seasonal variation and long-term bioaccumulation may occur in fish. The ratio of animal concentration to environmental concentration of cesium-137 has been estimated at five to one for mollusks, 20 to one for fish, and 25 to one for crustaceans.

Overall, in considering the activity of radionuclides in the food chain, three basic characteristics relevant to food safety management are apparent. The first is that the degree and type of radionuclides vary. In any radionuclide contamination, the degree and type will vary across geographic areas, among species, among individual animals within species, and over time. Some of this variability—in particular, variability between species and geographic areas—is predictable, at least in its broad outlines, based on rainfall at the time the contaminated cloud passes over, soil type, plant type, and exposure of animals to contaminated pasture or feeds. In Sweden, radioactivity in sheep after Chernobyl varied from below detectable limits (2 Bq/kg) to over 3.9 kBq/kg, in reindeer from 12 Bq/kg to over 16,000 Bq/kg, and in some species of fish from below detectable limits to 48,000 Bq/kg.

If we based our sampling for cesium-137 levels on the data from Sweden, and wished to be within 10 percent of the true average value 95 percent of the time, we would need about 200 milk samples, 1,000 beef samples, and some 400,000 reindeer. The Canadian government's 1986 report on radioactivity in Canada mentioned testing one caribou. For animals in which individual levels vary widely, such as fish and wildlife, simple random sampling to within a specified accuracy is probably impractical. A more focused sampling plan, based on expected hot spots, would yield more precise estimates based on fewer samples.

Second, radionuclides tend to be mobile. They do not just go to one place and sit; they move around in the ecosystem, influencing and being influenced by a myriad of biophysical parameters. Some of the key influential environmental factors have been identified: the amount of the competing stable element (potassium, iodine, calcium, etc), soil type (clay versus sand), water intake of plants (surface versus deep root), and feeding habits of animals (browsing versus grazing, close-cropping versus high-cropping, carnivorous versus herbivorous). These factors can be used to make initial decisions about both monitoring and food restrictions in a disaster.

Third, several of the radionuclides might be potentially concentrated as they move up through the levels of the food chain, particularly in aquatic systems. In other systems, radionuclides may be screened out. The concentration of iodine-131 in milk, for instance, is usually only a tenth of that of the vegetation consumed by the cow.

In responding to a nuclear crisis such as Chernobyl, a great deal of cooperation between farmers, veterinarians, food processors, and public health officials is required to ensure a reasonably safe food supply.

At the farm, both preventive and therapeutic actions are possible. Animals in a contaminated area should be kept indoors and fed stored, clean feeds. Where this is not possible—for instance, in some northern areas where animals are herded or hunted—hay could be transported from clean areas to specified feeding spots. After Chernobyl, some farmers attempted to decontaminate pastures by sending in sacrificial clean-up sheep. These animals were supposed to eat all of the contaminated plants and would then be killed. This tactic only works if the radioactivity stays in the leaves and stems; in many cases, it can be quickly relocated to roots. In that case, no amount of grazing will get rid of it. Clearly, with the high contamination rates noted earlier in sheep in both Norway and the United Kingdom in 2006, this strategy for decontamination was not very successful. In the reindeer-lichen ecosystem, the long effective half-life of radioactive elements needs to be balanced against the fact that the lichens do not have any root uptake. The clean-up grazing might work but, as God is reputed to have said to chances of peace in the Middle East, maybe not in my lifetime.

Some Swedish sheep farmers have pastured their animals in forested areas. The umbrella effect is only sometimes helpful, however; many plants that grow in the nutrient-poor soils of a coniferous forest are very efficient at accumulating available resources, including the contaminants we put into the system. This would seem to be the case, for instance, with the Norwegian sheep in 2006.

In the longer term, working lime- and potassium-rich fertilizers into the soil to act as stable competitors against the radionuclides and cutting grass down to 150-millimeters stubble have been reputed to decrease the radionuclide concentration in forages from contaminated areas. Tilling the soil after contamination but before planting pushes the cesium-137 down to root level, where uptake is lower than at the surface.

Individual animals can be decontaminated by feeding them chelating agents such as Prussian blue or bentonite, which attach to cesium in the intestine and prevent its absorption, or feeds high in potassium to compete for absorption with the cesium. If strontium-90 is present, high-calcium feeds such as legumes are appropriate. While cesium-137 may have a long physical half-life, animals in a clean environment on clean feed may be made safe by taking advantage of the relatively short biological half-life. The success of these actions depends in part on the removal of affected animals from the contaminated ecosystem and prompt therapy.

Plants from sandy soils, and those with shallow root systems that depend on surface moisture, such as mushrooms, and green, leafy plants that are in full leaf at the time of contamination, should be avoided for both animal and human consumption. Fruits and vegetables that can be peeled could perhaps be salvaged. Mature root crops, particularly in clay soils, are also less likely to be contaminated.

For people, milk and milk products provide the major route of exposure to iodine-131 and strontium-90. Meat is the major vehicle for exposure to cesium-137. When decisions are made about allocating resources and setting priorities, foods of animal origin might be ranked in decreasing order of suspicion— from small ruminants to beef cattle to dairy cattle to pigs and poultry. Within each of these categories, animals raised in total confinement can be separated out, and those with access to pasture can be targeted for special consideration. In the period shortly after the contamination, iodine-131 would be the major consideration. Later, cesium (and strontium) in both milk and meat would become the primary focus. As mentioned previously, storage of contaminated cheese is associated with the disappearance of radioactive iodine but with the concentration of radiocesium; testing of cheese before storage or disposal is therefore important.

Finally, it is all very well to say that we will dispose of contaminated foods—but how? After the Chernobyl disaster, the papers periodically unearthed stories of radioactive European chocolate being shipped to, say, Malaysia. Industrialized countries have been exporting wars and garbage and contaminants to the developing world for so long and with such impunity that I should not be surprised. I attended a talk by a Soviet scientist (when there still were Soviet scientists) on food safety after Chernobyl. He kept talking about disposing of radioactive milk. When I asked him what he meant by disposing, he hesitated just long enough for a very aggressive colleague of his—who perhaps had seen too many American movies about KGB agents and didn't wish to disappoint his audience—to step in and basically tell me that things were properly taken care of. I never did get a straight answer. A European colleague tells me that some of the contaminated food was simply recycled back into the system as food shortages developed.

Monitoring programs need to be tailored not only to the animals that are most likely to be contaminated but also to specific consumption patterns of the human population.

Milk needs to be carefully monitored, because it is a primary food source for children, who consume far more per unit of body weight than adults in the same society. Mothers' breast milk is safe, but only if the mother has not been exposed; about 20 percent of iodine-131 ingested by the mother can show up in the breast milk. Most of the contamination occurs in the first twelve hours after exposure. If not enough food has been prepared and stored before contamination, or if food supplies are doubtful, children and pregnant women should receive priority access to what safe food is available; having many actively growing tissues, they are acutely vulnerable to the effects of radionuclides.

Contamination of caribou or reindeer with radiocesium may be a more serious public health risk in some populations than the same levels in, say, cattle. People who eat beef not only tend to consume it as a small part of a voluminous diet but also usually have several other dietary alternatives available, while those who eat caribou have fewer choices and may use the meat as a more central part of their diet. It seems to make sense, strictly based on health, to set tolerance levels lower for major components of the diet and to provide alternative supplements to those who rely heavily on single food sources. Marine animals may provide one relatively safe alternative food source for people in contaminated northern areas. In general, it is logical to use fish near the top of the food chain during the early period after the disaster, before the radionuclides have an opportunity to work their way up through the system. Provided that the contamination was a one-time event, smaller fish near the bottom of the food chain would be expected to be safer later on.

Setting of tolerance levels for food will always be controversial in a crisis, and human health must always be defined beyond the reductionist framework of specifically measured radionuclides. The social consequences of some courses of action may have more devastating health effects than others. Biologically, a zero-tolerance level is untenable, either for domestic or imported foods, because of the universal presence of background radiation and the variation in risk for different foods and different population groups. Zero-tolerance regulations are based on the common misconception that it is possible to eat without risk.

In Sweden, action levels for contamination of foods after the Chernobyl accident were set at 300 Bq/kg in general and 1,500 Bq/kg for wild plants and animals. While this may be appropriate for urban southerners for whom wild-caught food is a small part of the diet, it may be totally inappropriate for certain northern or native populations.

Recommendations developed by the World Health Organization and the International Commission on Radiological Protection can serve as a starting point. Nevertheless, we need to avoid the fallacy of thinking that what is average should be the norm. This fallacy tends to protect some parts of the population beyond the bounds of common sense while leaving others, often cultural minorities and particularly vulnerable subgroups in the population, open to serious exposure. A more rational and reasonable approach would be to focus both monitoring and preventive programs on identified high-risk foods and vulnerable consumers.

In a crisis, decisions often have to be made based on "best judgments." In the end, we need to ask ourselves if the risks we take are necessary and if those who suffer are the same as those who benefit. What Chernobyl taught us is not only that what goes around comes around, but also that our responses to energy wants and climate change have implications for our food safety when the inevitable accident happens. Big nuclear plants may be cheaper and cleaner than coal plants, but the consequences of mistakes are also much bigger and harder to fix. There is, according to the old adage beloved (and interpreted differently) by economists and ecologists alike, no free lunch.

SPICING UP

THE

LONG-TERM

COMMITMENT

14

RISKS,
RIGHTS, AND
RIGHTEOUS
EATING

REVISITING RISK

CHAPTER 9 introduced the notion of risk assessment, which is the framework that scientists have been using since the 1990s to organize a variety of messy ideas about feelings of danger, and to put them on a measurable scientific footing. That chapter suggested that this framework can be useful but that there are a whole lot of things that fall between the cracks in the move from feelings to measurement. In this chapter, I want to uncover some of those losses and to see how they might inform us and maybe give us a richer, more realistic, and sustainable set of possibilities for dealing with the delicious and dangerous dilemmas facing us as we stare at our dinner plates.

The scientific idea of risk is one of probabilities and includes the notion that the event being considered is an unfavorable one. Thus, the World Health Organization defines risk as an expected frequency of undesirable effects arising from exposure to something. We may think of risk as the rate of disease or death that occurs, or would occur, in a population exposed to a particular harmful agent. In general terms, we are all at risk for getting *Staph* poisoning, and we can attach a particular number to that (so many cases per million of population).

This way of expressing risk is based on reported numbers of cases of particular diseases in particular populations. This type of risk is not to be confused with the risks people talk about when they discuss chemicals in foods. Risk assessments are value judgments based on scientific estimates of what we think might happen; that is why they are always so controversial.

Risk, for most scientists, is measurable and abstract, a probability that is applied to a population. Risk, for each of us, is personal and immediate, an outcome applied to me. I feel it as danger. Minimizing risks at a population level may result in higher risks for certain individuals. How can notions of individual risks and population risks be reconciled? Let me work through several examples.

One disease that resonates in the public mind across these complicated and contradictory layers is bovine spongiform encephalopathy (BSE), popularly referred to as mad cow disease.

In 1986, a new neurological disease was recognized in British cattle, characterized by slow onset, changed behavior (fear or aggression), incoordination, falling, tremors, and abnormal responses to touch and sound. The brains of the diseased cattle looked like sponges. They also looked like brains of sheep that had died of a disease called scrapie, as well as like the brains of people who had died from such very rare diseases as Creuzfeldt-Jakob disease, fatal familial insomnia, and kuru; like the brains of mink that had died from transmissible mink encephalopathy, and like the brains of deer and elk that had died of chronic wasting disease in the North American Midwest. These diseases are called, as a group, transmissible spongiform encephalopathies (that is, transmissible spongelike brain degeneration). But transmissible by what? Most of these diseases—except for chronic wasting disease in parts of North America—are very rare, so they are difficult to study. How might they be transmitted?

Sporadic Creuzfeldt-Jakob (the "traditional" form of the disease) does not appear to be infectious, but it occurs so rarely (maybe one in a million people get it) that this is difficult to study. On the one hand, the fact that it is so rare seems to suggest that it is not infectious. On the other hand, the fact that Creuzfeldt-Jakob disease has been transmitted with corneal transplants, grafts of dura mater (the tissue that covers the brain), and surgical contamination suggests that it can be *transmitted*. So what is transmissible that is not infectious?

During the BSE epidemic, cases were reported in house cats and cats in zoos (but not in dogs given the same diet). Could it jump to people? The epidemic of the new disease in British cattle peaked at several thousand cases per month in the early 1990s, after which government initiatives to stop the recycling of dead ruminant offal began to have their effects.

The first transmissible spongiform encephalopathy of people to be described was kuru, investigated by a veterinarian working with the South Fore people of New Guinea, which is the only place in the world where it occurs. The word "kuru" means "shivering" in the local language; people who came down with the disease suffered a gradual loss of body control. At first, they may have appeared merely clumsy, stumbling and falling over. This symptom progressed to tremors and twitches, shivering, and then, eventually, immobilization and death. Mostly women and children were affected; they got to eat the brains and nervous tissue of people who had died, while the men got the muscle. The disease did not appear to be infectious.

Was the new disease in cows infectious? If not, how did it spread? If so, could people get it by eating meat? Amid the wave of public fear and general uncertainty (not the most ideal conditions for a cool scientific assessment), epidemiologist John Wilesmith explored every possible option. One theory has been that the disease crossed the species barrier from sheep into cattle. Another is that it was always present at a low level in cattle and that rendering and recycling practices simply magnified what was already there. In general, the story that emerged from the work of Wilesmith and his colleagues was complicated, disconcerting, and humbling.

In agriculture, efficiency is the name of the game. Efficiency, the art and practice of not wasting anything, keeps prices down. When animals are raised for meat, there is potentially a lot of "waste." I put this word in quotation marks because in natural systems, there is no waste. Animals that die become food for trees, for insects, for fungi. Nothing is wasted in nature. Waste is a concept related to human use. Anything we can't use for ourselves is considered waste. In the livestock industry, animals get sick; at slaughter there are parts of animals that don't appear to have immediate human use, at least in European or North American culture. Looked at another way, however, all this waste is good protein and energy. Young animals that get protein and energy supplements grow faster. One might call this the hamburger effect: North American kids are taller than their parents, even if the parents are from Japan or China, and a lot of what we once thought was genetic has now been shown to be dietary.

One way to keep the price of meat products down is to recycle all those parts of slaughtered animals that are considered unfit for human consumption and feed them back to the livestock as protein supplements. This practice is terribly efficient. On the face of it, it even seems "green." Isn't recycling good?

Rendering plants recycle dead animals back into the animal food chain by converting animal offal into fat (tallow) and defatted meat and bone meal (MBM to insiders) to be used in animal

feeds. Trade in these products is huge—hundreds of millions of dollars' worth annually, going to and coming from just about every country in the world. This is global ecology writ large, and it is largely invisible to just about everyone except those who are directly involved. If you search the web, you will find that this kind of recycling falls into a general category that may include not just meat and bonemeal but also poultry meal, organic fertilizer, animal fat, used tires, and plastic scraps. Recycling is good business.

Until the late 1970s, rendering plants in the United Kingdom utilized energy-hungry processes that involved mixing, steam-heating, milling, and extraction of fat using hydrocarbon organic products. In the 1970s, fuel prices increased, some animal production managers began to prefer more fat in the feed, and industries became concerned that worker health and safety were threatened by the old processes. So the processes were changed and the hydrocarbon extraction process was dropped, as were processing temperatures.

The United Kingdom has millions of sheep, many of which die before the food system can kill them. Before the emergence of BSE, the remains of these sheep were recycled as feed for other animals. Scrapie, a mysterious, madly itching disease in which sheep scrape off their wool against whatever surface they can find, was endemic in the United Kingdom sheep population at about 2 percent. Farmers and veterinarians have known about scrapie since the 1700s, and, although sheep could clearly pass it one to another, there had never been any hint that it could be passed to other species.

Pathologists had identified strange proteins in the brains of sheep infected with scrapie; they were called prions. In the 1970s, when I was going through veterinary college, the accepted wisdom about scrapie was that (1) prions could not cause the disease because they didn't have any DNA or RNA as bacteria and viruses do, and (2) diseases like scrapie would not jump between species. In 1997, Stanley Prusiner, who demonstrated that malformed prions do indeed cause a range of diseases by transforming normal proteins they come in contact with, and that they can cross species barriers, received a Nobel Prize for his work. That this change in the opinions of (most) scientists took place after much debate, some of it rancorous, can be attributed both to the difficult personalities of some of the people involved, and the basic principle that, if a scientist makes an assertion that goes against our best understanding of the way the world works, that scientist's work is subject to very intense scrutiny. There is a lot at stake here. If I say that a certain river flows downhill, or that a particular bacterium causes disease, or that pesticides cause mad cow disease, my observations do not put into question whole bodies of scholarship. If I assert that a river flows uphill, or that a normal protein with no known means of reproduction causes disease, I am either slightly crazy, or I have made a profound new discovery. That this change of opinion took place at all can be attributed both to the dogged persistence of the investigators involved, and, ultimately, to the openness of science to new evidence.

If the BSE investigators had read more widely, thought more laterally, and understood better that nature always surprises, they might have considered not just kuru and scrapie but also chronic wasting disease. First identified in captive mule deer in Colorado in the 1960s, this is a fatal prion disease of white-tailed deer (*Odocoileus virginiatus*), Rocky Mountain elk (*Cervus elaphus nelsoni*) and mule deer (*Odocoileus hemionus*). Like scrapie, but unlike some other prion diseases, chronic wasting disease seems to cluster and to be spread from animal to animal. Investigators have found it in farmed and wild deer. It has been spread by movements of farmed animals, and it appears to have traveled and spread among animals in the wild; it may be spread through feces and saliva. In deer, the clinical signs range from lack of coordination, separation from the herd, and weight loss to pneumonia and increases in drinking and urinating. Animals take weeks to months to die, which all afflicted animals do. Can hunters get it? I could say, facetiously, that it depends what you eat. But this is not a disease to be facetious about. Scientists don't know.

Scientists now think that there are multiple strains of prions and can differentiate cattle prions from sheep prions from people prions and so on. Everyone has normal prions in his or her nervous tissues. There is some evidence that, for some of the prion diseases, such as chronic wasting disease and scrapie, the prions may be in the muscles as well as the nervous tissue, especially if the animal has more than one infection concurrently. There is also some evidence that, like rabies viruses, infectious prions can travel down the nerves to the salivary gland. Malformed prions—the ones that cause disease—are really, really hard to destroy.

In 1994, the first cases of what was called variant Creuzfeldt-Jakob disease appeared. The disease is similar to sporadic Creuzfeldt-Jakob disease but more painful and longer lasting (average fourteen months of illness versus four months) and strikes younger people (average age of onset twenty-nine years versus sixty years). The good news is that the disease is also not easily transmitted. So far, only a couple of hundred cases of variant Creuzfeldt-Jakob disease have showed up in the United Kingdom, despite the many opportunities for people to have been exposed to BSE prions.

The gaps in our knowledge about these diseases are very large. We are uncertain about the meaning of what we do know. Philosophers of science Silvio Funtowicz and Jerry Ravetz point out that in situations characterized by uncertainties and conflicts in ethics and knowledge, the scientific evidence is "soft," and the policy decisions are hard, which is the reverse of what our society has come to expect or desire. Funtowicz and Ravetz have called for a new kind of publicly engaged science, which

202 · FOOD, SEX, AND SALMONELLA

they call postnormal science. I'll come back to that later, but the transmissible spongiform encephalopathies surely represent just such a situation.

In 1988, at a conference in Ottawa, John Wilesmith, a vibrant young epidemiologist, was lionized as a new John Snow, one of the great ninteenth-century practitioners of epidemiology, who had discovered that water transmitted cholera in London and halted the epidemic by removing a pump handle. Like Snow, Wilesmith and his colleagues had carried out well-designed, well-executed, elegant studies on the causes of the epidemic of mad cow disease. I saw him again in 1998, in Paris, after a decade of harassment from politicians and a public demanding certainty, puffing on a cigarette and looking broken down and tired (more perhaps like a living great-grandfather of epidemiology).

I was reminded of a story told by Robert Desowitz, a parasitologist who for many years worked with the World Health Organization, in his book *New Guinea Tapeworms and Jewish Grandmothers*. One of the tribal groups in what is now Irian Jaya suffered from many serious incidents of cerebral cysticercosis associated with our old friend, the tapeworm *Taenia solium*. Occasionally, these worms will, in an act of capitalist ingenuity, rebel against the boring old human intestinal job description and strike out adventurously into the circuitous channels of the body. Some of them, rafting the channels to the brain, get stuck there, where they make home and havoc. Victims in Irian Jaya would be thrown into convulsions and often fall into the fire, where they were severely burned. The tapeworm came to these people, ironically, through an appeasement present of Balinese pigs from the president of Indonesia after annexation.

After Desowitz made some frustrating attempts to persuade the people to cook their meat well, the chief told him that to prevent the disease the people would have to change deeply ingrained cultural habits. Having already lost much control over their lives to the Indonesian invaders, however, they were not now about to give up this last vestige of their self-esteem just to stay healthy. The Indonesian governor later remarked to Desowitz on the primitiveness and stubbornness of these people, who did not want to make minor changes in their behavior to improve their health. Desowitz was about to agree when he noticed that he and the governor were both smoking cigarettes.

I am sure that Wilesmith knew about the risks associated with smoking, but he would also have known that those risks are based on probabilities and apply to populations. People who smoke are more likely to get lung cancer; that's an irrefutable population fact. Individuals who smoke may nonetheless thrill at the sense of danger and take comfort in the possibility of beating the odds. I don't know what Wilesmith was feeling or thinking. He may even have felt a sadness at being addicted, enslaved to a large corporation not much different from a large totalitarian government. For some factory workers, a smoke break may be the only time in a day when a factory worker can *feel* free, even if, as Leonard Cohen said, that freedom might look to others like death. In a sense, the contradictory forces that characterize the tobacco-use debate (social obsessions, "addictions" to certain foods or ideas, individual rights, and public responsibilities) are not so much different from those that gave rise to the BSE epidemic.

If BSE gave steak an aura of danger, then several other organisms have done the same for raw milk.

In the 1980s, some Canadian government scientists floated a proposal that cheese made from unpasteurized milk be banned. For cheese lovers of south European and Latin descent, this suggestion was seen as an attack on their culture. The organism that the government scientists were concerned about, *Listeria monocytogenes,* can be found widely in the environment—in water, soil, vegetation, sewage, and the intestines of healthy animals and people. As a veterinarian, I was taught that this organism was the cause of a rare condition in cattle, called circling disease, which occurred as the result of an abscess in the brain. The cows, so the story went, picked it up from poorly prepared silage, a kind of bovine version of sauerkraut.

Before the 1980s, listeriosis in people was rarely reported and was not particularly associated with food. The disease appeared as abortion, blood infections, and infections of the nervous system. It was once thought to affect only immunocompromised people. In the 1980s, that pattern seemed to change. The infection, which could be associated with a transient gut problem, is now known to be more common than investigators had suspected. Although infection is common, and disease is rare, almost a third of those who get the disease die. How does one calculate an acceptable risk? When is it appropriate for the food-consuming public to feel anxious, to sense danger, and, hence, for the authorities to regulate?

In Los Angeles in 1985, 142 people got sick and forty-eight died, many of them babies. The source was a Mexican-style soft cheese that included some unpasteurized milk. A smaller outbreak was associated with the same product in North Carolina in 2000. During the 1990s, outbreaks of listeriosis in Europe were reportedly associated with cheese, pork tongue in jelly, and some fish products. These outbreaks, and a report from the Centers for Disease Control and Prevention in Atlanta that some people were getting it from ready-to-eat hot dogs, sent a panic through the food industry. Investigators began looking everywhere for the bug and, not surprisingly, given its cosmopolitan living habits, began finding it everywhere.

As critics of the Canadian government proposal pointed out, the first foodborne outbreak of listeriosis was not associated with cheese at all. During a six-month period in 1981, in the Canadian Maritime provinces, an epidemic of listeriosis affected forty-one people, a third of whom, mostly newborn infants, died. This Canadian epidemic was traced to commercially prepared coleslaw. The coleslaw was made using cabbage that had been fertilized with manure from sheep, some of which had suffered from clinical listeriosis.

Listeria monocytogenes (like the appendicitis-mimicking *Yersinia*, mentioned in chapter 2), thrives in cool temperatures, so the cold-storage procedures and refrigeration associated with cabbages and coleslaw provided a perfect environment. The same can be said for ready-to-eat foods like wieners and cheeses, especially those non-aged white cheeses like Camembert and Mexican white cheese. In other words, refrigeration, which we use to protect us against most foodborne illnesses, allows *Listeria* to grow.

Drinking unpasteurized milk is a risky business. The barnyard, and indeed the udder itself, is a veritable United Nations of bacteria with names like *Yersinia, Listeria, E. coli, Campylobacter,* and *Salmonella.* In the old days, and even now in rural communities, many farm families drink their milk straight. They may even offer some to the veterinarian who lives just down the road. Many people who drink this raw milk have done so for years and claim it tastes better than pasteurized milk. A student doing a project with the Perth County health unit in Ontario decided to test this claim. Her parents drink raw milk, they said, because of the flavor. One day, she surreptitiously started pasteurizing it for them, and they never detected the difference. Our perception of taste is dramatically influenced by what goes on in our minds.

Some people also claim that raw milk is better for you. How can this veritable staff of life make us sick? In the 1980s, one medical officer of health in our area told me that farm families were usually loath to change their ways and get a home pasteurizer until their kids ended up in the hospital attached to intravenous tubes. She reported that in her county, rates of clinical disease from *Salmonella, Campylobacter,* and *Yersinia* were much higher in farm families who drank raw milk than in city dwellers. A lifetime of drinking raw milk will endow the imbibers—those that survive—with a certain resistance to the bacteria therein. Hence we often hear the condescending comment, accompanied by a chuckle, "Well, my grandfather drank it for seventy years."

Grandpa, who drank that milk all his life, does not remember his childhood ailments so clearly any more; nor does he connect milk with the little brother who died at the age of two from some mysterious ailment. But if we could go back and carefully sort through all those so-called "stomach flu" problems that plague every childhood, we would find that some of them were caused by VTEC, or *Salmonella, Campylobacter, Yersinia,* or some of the hundreds of other invisible bugs that share the barnyard with the more photogenic bipeds and quadrupeds.

Consumers in North America and Europe are fortunate that dairy farmers have largely, but not completely, eradicated tuberculosis and brucellosis, two of the more serious diseases that consumed raw-cow-milk drinkers in the "good old days." Goats in southern Europe still carry the most serious form of brucellosis, and goats and sheep everywhere still carry another serious disease, Q fever.

Milk, it should be said, is food for baby cows, not baby people. By stealing the cream from another species' crop, humanity is not only cleverly outcompeting other species but also endangering itself. Certainly, pasteurization can be a way of "laundering the money" in a centralized food system. Large-scale milk production and distribution would not be safely possible without pasteurization; by the same token, the capital investments necessary for pasteurization (at least for certain kinds of pasteurizers), as for many other food safety technologies, require a large throughput of material to be economically viable. Thus, the technology itself reinforces the tendency to move to economies of scale and tends to push smaller (often organic) producers to the margins, if not out of business altogether. In this way, economic power is centralized and society is deprived of real choice in food sources. I would call this economic "de-democratization." So, to the extent that pasteurization is used as an excuse to centralize and de-democratize our eating, we need to put on some cautionary brakes.

But that is not the whole story. It's one thing to share the goods all in the family, but if we are going to offer to feed the world with it, we need to take precautions. Milk is good, nutritionally, for that minority of us in the world who can digest it. Not everyone wants or likes or needs milk. My mother-in-law, raised in China, says that her Chinese playmates would talk about how the Europeans smelled offensively sour, like cheese. Being of good Germanic stock, I do love my milk and cheese and full-cream ice cream, but I have been on enough dairy farms to know better than to indulge promiscuously.

The chief justification for drinking and distributing raw milk is a philosophical and ideological one: that people should be able to drink what they please without the interference of the state. I have considerable sympathy for this skeptical view of state reasonableness. Again, it comes back to a mixture of science and values.

In an attempt to balance the public good with individual preference, some parts of North America have created certification programs for sellers of raw milk. The certification process is supposed to ensure that the farm and milk are clean. A clean farm and healthy animals are no guarantee of bacteriological safety, however; many of the organisms of most concern from a public health viewpoint cause few problems in animals. In one *Salmonella* epidemic in a large veterinary hospital, the bacteria were hiding in the soap trays at the sinks! Hiding right under— or, for bacteria, in—the detective's nose is a trick that goes all the way back to the bacterial soup we emerged from a billion or two years ago. Cows can leak *Listeria* out in their milk and *E. coli* O157:H7 in their manure without looking sick.

208 · FOOD, SEX, AND SALMONELLA

We also know, from outbreaks, that pasteurized milk is associated with foodborne disease outbreaks. What do we do with this information? Regulators have often focused on unpasteurized milk as a danger because it has been associated with many other diseases, and we have a readily available technology to make the milk "safe."

Furthermore, my arguments on pasteurization as a centralizing technology notwithstanding, unlike, say, irradiation, pasteurization need not necessitate centralization, even though it has often been used to do so. Home pasteurizers are available, and some research is being done on the use of microwaves to kill the pathogens in milk. It thus passes one of the most crucial tests for appropriate technology: its social effects are malleable and reversible. Nevertheless, I expect that reasonable people may disagree with me on this.

We are left pondering systemic issues, embedded in social-ecological systems—the uneven spread of risk through the system, the possible terrible dangers for some people and happy benefits for others. Because individual acts and collective parties are linked in a variety of feedback loops, problems of individual choice, food safety, agricultural practice, obesity, efficiency, and global trade cannot be simply resolved, in isolation from each other, by some scientific or technological sleight of hand.

Creuzfeldt-Jakob disease is a terrible, fatal affliction for the individuals who get it. Yet the risk (probability) of getting the variant Creuzfeldt-Jakob disease in the United Kingdom (the country with the most cases) is at most around three per million, which is about the same as the risk of getting listeriosis in Canada. At the height of the epidemic of BSE in England, Peter Gzowski, an interviewer on the Canadian Broadcasting Corporation, asked me if I would eat a steak from England, if he threw it on the barbecue and invited me over for supper. I said yes, I would, because I valued his company.

Risk is not only unevenly distributed but can also change as quickly as our ideological and culinary whims. Consumers demand fresh or minimally processed foods, safe products, low prices, and fat-free, sugar-free foods that taste as if they contain fat and sugar. In response, producers and agrifood companies offer "modified atmosphere" technologies (to keep the food "fresh") that can alter the normal bacterial life on food in unforeseen and sometimes dangerous ways.

Eating habits of North Americans, and of the newly rich everywhere, have changed dramatically (mostly in favor of more meat and more eating out, often fatty foods) since the 1950s. Americans each eat about 190 pounds of (boneless) meat per year. Between 1970 and the mid-1990s, eating out went from about 25 percent of the household food budget to about 40 percent. The increases and changes in consumption have come at a time when these fatty overeaters need a lot fewer calories to get a day's work done. The costs of these changes in diabetes, heart disease, cancer, and just plain getting fat are huge—to the people affected, to the environment, to the medical and disease-care systems. At the other end of the scale are the people who produce and deliver the food. Most of the millions of people who gather the harvest, process the food, and serve it to consumers are poorly paid and poorly educated. They often lack job security, good toilet facilities, health care, or knowledge of hygiene. The globalization of the food supply has simply accentuated the fault lines that already existed in the agrifood system.

The risk for some groups of people relative to others is not only skewed by altered eating habits but also differentially distributed among age groups. Children show up in the foodborne illness reports more often than adults for various reasons. For one thing, Mom and Dad are more likely to take Baby to the doctor with the trots than if they get the trots. For another, infants are at risk for infant botulism because they lack a competitive intestinal flora, an inherent factor, and because they so aggressively sample their environmental bacteria, a behavioral factor. Children under nine years of age are reported with *Salmonella* and *Campylobacter* infections more often than adults, often because adults feed them foods, such as raw milk or flesh, for which their bodies are ill prepared. Children and older people may have less acidic stomachs, which make them more hospitable to bacterial visitors.

College students are another risky age group. This is a side effect of second weaning, when the kids leave home and begin to prepare their own foods, without many of the requisite skills. One study in the United States found that raw-oyster eaters were most likely to be males between eighteen and forty-nine years old who were cigarette smokers, drank a lot of alcohol, and reported drinking while driving. Risky behavior, it seems, comes in self-reinforcing lifestyle constellations. In this case, the clustering of behaviors was reinforced by the structure of the food-service industry (i.e., an oyster bar brings the high risks related to oysters, those related to alcohol, and those related to "bar" behavior together in one place).

Older people, particularly those who have chronic diseases, are on medications, or eat institutional food, are another age group at risk. The mass-produced food provides more opportunities for bacteria to enter and multiply; the people on antacids have stomachs that are more captive to those bacteria. In general, people who are debilitated from other diseases succumb more easily than healthy individuals to foodborne illness. Their bodies are already compromised, or at least too busy fighting on other fronts to even think about assaults from food. The proportion of immunocompromised people in the world has increased as a result of AIDS, cancer, cancer treatments, and a variety of other chronic conditions.

Risks are magnified through mass production systems. Cheese, organic vegetables, and noodles prepared for mass consumption cannot be thought of in the same mental breath as those prepared for the family at home. You can't take organic, small-scale production systems and simple ramp them up for the mass market. That's asking for disaster. It is one thing to put your friends at risk. It is quite another thing to put at risk consumers in general, a group that includes not only traditionally vulnerable groups such as pregnant women and young children but, more and more, substantial numbers of people with chronic and/or immunosuppressive disorders. One may have a right, for instance, to share unpasteurized milk with consenting adults, but does one have the right to put innocent children at risk?

Traditions that we value are not always a reliable guide in this complex new world. Our grandparents may not have recognized the risks associated with eating certain foods. Who among them would worry about a few cases of diarrhea or headaches? Who would know to blame the food? That might imply that Grandma did something wrong in the kitchen, and that was not something one implied with impunity. With so many children dying in infancy, one was happy just to have food and to survive. Some of the diseases we now recognize exist precisely because we can now recognize them. The background morbidity and mortality is washed away, the invisible invaders' magic potion has suddenly worn off, and there they are, naked as jaybirds, sitting and grinning hungry grins at the kitchen table.

Risk, then, is related to the food itself and to the nature of the people eating the food, to work habits, and to social conditions. The poor are more likely than others to lack clean water, buy low-grade, contaminated "cheap" cooking oil, or eat seeds treated with toxic fungicides. People who work in the kitchen, or those who make sausages, are exposed to raw foods, where millions of tiny living beings thrive. Farmers are more likely to drink raw milk than city people and hence to expose themselves quite blatantly to bacterial invaders. As one might imagine, slaughterhouse workers, laboring amid the sprays of blood and airborne flesh, are easy targets. Inuit and Indians may eat fermented whale meat, seal flippers, or raw bear meat. Menno-nites may make meat buns together, Italians may prepare pasta communally, and Jews may express their togetherness by avoid-ing pork and indulging in gefilte fish. Belgian mothers nibble on raw ground pork. But these cooks go the gefilte fish makers one better: they share this delight with their children, introducing them not only to a great cultural tradition but also to *Y. entero-colitica*. Although Belgian researchers knew that mothers and children had the highest rates of disease, they decided that get-ting Belgians to change their ways in the kitchen was hopeless. The only way to control the disease was to attack the organism in the comfort of its porcine home; however, the suggestion that changing the microbial ecology in pig populations is easier, or less costly, than changing cultural habits is marked by a certain naivete, however. The less one knows about a subject, I suppose, the simpler it seems, and since so few people know about raising pigs, changing their bacterial ecology must be "easy," right? In the couple of decades since the suggestions were made, research-ers have explored sophisticated screening at slaughterhouses (so that infected lymph nodes could be trimmed out) and vaccines, but I don't expect to see the bacteria eradicated from pigs in my lifetime. Even if it were, as the case of *Salmonella pullorum* and *S. enteritidis* illustrates, nature would likely replace the missing *Yersinia* with something else, probably worse.

We also put ourselves into danger by personal decisions. Before my egg allergy set in, I used to eat homemade eggnog and hollandaise sauce, for instance, though I should have known better than to eat raw eggs. I recall sitting down with my backpack at a small Thai cafe in 1968 and asking for scrambled eggs; I was given raw eggs, scrambled in a glass, with soy sauce added. I drank it—as well as something called cholera juice made from mangoes and street water, in Calcutta, and lived to write a book about foodborne disease. It is naive to believe that nature protects the naive; for every survivor who lives to write books, there are many who have died.

The stories of BSE and listeriosis are typical of what has happened in the agrifood industry and raise some fundamental questions about hazards, risks, and how society manages them. If the risky agent is everywhere but only makes a few food consumers sick, should governments gear up the whole system to protect those few, or is it eater beware? Can society protect the ignorant or the stupid? Should it? If a child is fed raw milk by the parent and develops a serious disease, what is the responsibility of society? Should there be a special food section in the store for those who are young, pregnant, or immunocompromised? If recycling of biological material (manure, dead animals) results in recycling of bacteria, parasites, chemicals, or prions, what can we do?

Despite a wave of popular books arguing to the contrary, eating is more than bodily nourishment, and a meal is more than food. There are reasons why the algae grown on oil or bacteria grown in vats, promised to us as liberators from world hunger a decade ago, do not appeal to us. At a very basic level, we do eat for nourishment, of course—but what constitutes proper nourishment? Oat bran and raisins? Borscht and rollkuchen? Kingfish and rice? Noodles and tomato sauce? Hamburgers? Steak tartare? Puffer fish? Unpasteurized milk?

Eating is an essential ingredient in our understanding of ourselves, a literal coming to our senses. For this reason, eating is intimately bound up with our sense of being, individually and culturally. The food poisonings we suffer reflect not only hygiene and agricultural practices but, at a very deep level, who we are and who we are not. You can tell who a person is by what she chooses to make herself sick.

At a personal level, one way to deal with the problems of risk, and to reduce the sense of personal danger, is to identify those foods that pose the least risk and build one's diet around them. It seems, at first glance, to be a rational approach. This approach has often been married to a natural foods approach, that is, the eating of less-processed foods, which in general I favor. Nevertheless, the evangelical marriage of what is called natural eating, with a zealous attention to individual health, removes eating from its true ecological and social context. Through its oversimplifications, it can create as many problems as it solves.

The moral to be drawn is not that we avoid fresh foods but that eating broccoli or lettuce is not necessarily, taken out of context, a virtue. How are the farm workers who picked the lettuce being treated? Do they have good toilets? Time to go to them? Lots of water to wash their hands? Good medical facilities? Were they carrying hepatitis or parasites? Who prepared the food? Were they adequately educated in the fine arts of kitchen hygiene? Remember, you are about to become intimate with this salad. Do you know where it has been?

All of which brings me back to risks and dangers. Having acknowledged that children, pregnant women, and immuno-compromised people need special consideration, we are still left with eleven million Canadians, 76 million Americans, and a billion people worldwide getting sick from their food every year. Is our food putting us all at risk? Should we demand that it be perfectly safe?

Do I have a sense of danger when I am eating? That depends on where I am and with whom I am eating, but generally, no. I am more scared of the technocrats who are squabbling away our planetary future to protect economic or political or religious ideologies than I am of the food on my plate or the drink in my glass.

As this book should make clear, there are no firm answers to what constitutes a safe food or how we should regulate food safety. There's no silver bullet. Apart from the obvious and serious acute risks of bacteria and poisons that kill and maim outright, the riskiness of food is proper grist for the democratic mill. To suggest that food should be without risk or to believe that the food industry knows which risks are best for us and will take care of things is naive. The real questions in food safety are questions of values and ethics. The technical questions, by comparison, are trivial.

15

MONTEZUMA

RULES

THE

WORLD

DEAL WITH IT

A LONG THE Atlantic coast of Guatemala, the banana plantations of a couple of large U.S. food companies stretch from Guatemala south into Honduras, the country that gave the world the term "banana republic." Few people noticed the protests of banana plantation workers in the streets of Antigua during U.S. president Clinton's 1999 visit to Central America. Not newsworthy.

Who really wants to know about where their bananas come from, about massive restructuring of the landscape with earth movers, drains, and concrete, about the continuous use of pesticides, about the near-slavery of workers who are underpaid, overworked, and sprayed with banned pesticides? Bad for the markets, *that* news. A few disgruntled lefties might be aware of the 1954 overthrow of the democratically elected government in Guatemala by the United States to protect those banana plantation owners and the 1999 trade war with Europe to protect the interests of those same companies. Farther inland, along the winding roads, there are vast fields covered with fine mesh nets where so-called nontraditional export crops are grown: broccoli, snow peas, whatever is in fashion in the United States and Canada. One farmer told me that they were competing with several African countries to keep their costs down, and it was getting more difficult every year.

And what does any of this have to do with food safety? Although bananas and broccoli do not rank high in the annals of foodborne illness, they do represent the ways in which North Americans and Europeans think about risk. Scientists from the wealthy, industrialized parts of the world measure risk according to probabilities that consumers will get sick. In many cases, the result is that risks are simply shifted from consumers in wealthy importing countries to the poor farmers in exporting countries. The consumers get cheap bananas and veggies; the banana growers get pesticide toxicity, job uncertainty, and environmental degradation. I'll come back to this specifically with regard to the *Cyclospora* in raspberries a bit later in this chapter.

The emergence and spread of foodborne illnesses described in this book are not part of a plot from the left or the right. There have been a few cases of deliberate "bioterrorism" related to food, but they are not discussed in this book, because focusing on them gives all the wrong messages about where the big dangers are.

The pandemics and epidemics and outbreaks of *Salmonella* and other diseases are simply the natural outcomes of the logic of the marketplace, the logical conclusions of our lowest-prices-in-town agrifood system, the end result of my shopping preferences for healthy food in a supermarket. Changes in agricultural practices since 1945 have been driven almost exclusively by the goal to produce large volumes of low-cost food. With a dramatically increasing world population, a large proportion of whom live in poverty, this is an important goal. But the gains have been accompanied by problems, some of them serious and some of them surprising, suggesting that we need new ways of thinking about agriculture and other such activities. The *Cyclospora* outbreaks in North America traced back to Guatemala are a message about the state of the system. Are we listening? Are we looking at the evidence?

Agricultural production has increased largely by using methods based on standard experimental techniques and relatively simple linear cause-and-effect models. In the 1980s, building on the success of this linear, predict-and-control thinking, food safety specialists introduced Hazard Analysis Critical Control Points, or HACCP (pronounced hassip). HACCP is a simple set of guidelines stating that we should identify potential hazards to our food, note the critical points for preventing their entry into our food or for controlling them, implement controls, and monitor those points. Unlike some older methods of food safety, which relied on spot checks to determine whether food was contaminated, HACCP ensures that the processes through which foods pass on their way from the farm to the fork are based on scientific evidence for avoiding or eliminating or reducing hazards.

HACCP has become a buzzword in the food industry worldwide, largely because of a childlike delight some American regulators have taken in it. This delight has raised a great deal of suspicion among some consumer groups, who see HACCP as a way for large companies to justify high-volume, fast movement of animals through slaughterhouses and poor inspection of slaughterhouses with high profits. But proponents argue that this need not be the case. Because the only serious foodborne disease problems, whether chemical or bacterial, are invisible, it makes no sense to have a food inspection system that relies on visual appraisal of every item. Scientifically based sampling and testing do make sense, but we need to be vigilant and build in proper social safeguards.

The application of HACCP procedures from farm to fork, as the food industry is wont to say, is at best problematic. If applied broadly and carefully enough by identifying hazards as weaknesses in the overall food production and distribution system and not just technical or bacterial problems, this system could be used to help us change the whole agrifood system. The problem is that HACCP is based on a worldview that works pretty well in a factory, slaughterhouse, food-processing plant, or fast food restaurant, but it is a crummy system for dealing with the complex entanglements of the real world of food, where environmental sustainability, cultural food practices, public health, and economic viability all interact at various scales (household to globe) and are interpreted by a variety of people. Individual farmers make production decisions, national and other authorities set economic and political incentives, and regional or global market pressures reflect transnational corporate initiatives. Consumers make decisions based on personal and cultural histories and economic circumstances.

The patterns of foodborne disease reflect the dynamics of self-organizing systems. While conscious human choices play important roles in these systems, they are usually based on immediate considerations and do not recognize many secondary implications, much less overall system effects. No one controls the patterns formed when these choices and their effects combine. Few people are even aware of the patterns.

Not surprisingly, unintended consequences are both common and difficult to trace. Typically, they occur at one scale and from one perspective (e.g., that of an individual raspberry eater who gets sick) but are the result of decisions made from another perspective and at another scale (e.g., by government officials drafting regional economic policy). Moreover, the usual solutions developed for one set of narrowly defined problems (e.g., food production, food availability, or personal health) often create the sufficient conditions for another set of problems to emerge (e.g., ecological degradation and the emergence of infectious diseases).

In almost all cases where agricultural actions negatively affect health and the environment, individual farmers are making production decisions in response to economic and political incentives coming from a higher level—usually national governments—which themselves are responding to regional or global pressures. Usually, these effects are uni-directional—that is, farmers respond fairly quickly to global markets, which respond sluggishly, if at all, to changes in local farming conditions. Because agriculture is as profoundly ecological as it is economical in nature, the production decisions have biological effects that are local and often environmentally destructive, to which farmers have difficulty responding because of the socio-economic context in which they work. Due to the globalization of agriculture and the adaptability of micro-organisms, however, diseases such as salmonellosis, cyclosporiasis, and bovine spongiform encephalopathy serve as messages of system dysfunction coming through feedback links that have been blocked politically and economically.

If a farmer produces certain crops for consumption by his or her own family, the links between the production system and land degradation, water use, or foodborne disease are clear, and the farmer can quickly adjust how he or she grows and prepares the food. As production increases, and the webs of trade encompass a wider geographic range, such feedback becomes increasingly difficult. If the food is grown and distributed within one political jurisdiction (a province, a state, a country), the farmer might still make adjustments in a timely fashion. When, as the result of political and economic policies, food is grown in large monocultures, sent through distribution centers, and distributed globally, the feedback loops are sluggish and fragmented.

By the time the message at one end of the trail (foodborne disease in the consumer, land degradation on the farm) makes its way back to the place where it might influence practices, the farmer is out of business or the consumer has switched to other foods. In fact, in many cases, the foods cannot even be traced from "farm to fork," and the feedback loops are lost entirely.

Foodborne illnesses are the voice of nature. Are we listening? And if we listen, what do we hear? One problem is that each actor in the drama interprets the story differently.

Let us reconsider the issue of parasites in Guatemalan raspberries. A Guatemalan farmer might identify the following elements as being important: a third to two-thirds of the children in the country are malnourished, about three-quarters of the population lives in extreme poverty, the country has a foreign debt of over US$2.5 billion, and about 78 percent of the farms are marginalized by wealthy landowners to 10 percent of the land. From this point of view, the problem is not one of parasites on raspberries, which are a trivial issue in the global context of serious diseases; probably half the cases of cyclosporiasis in the United States are unrelated to imported raspberries, and many tons of raspberries were shipped to the United States (especially during the autumn harvest peak) that did not cause problems.

The problem from the point of view of poor Guatemalan farmers is how to create sustainable livelihoods from a very small land base that is rapidly degrading. Without major land distribution or social reorganization, it appears that the cash to buy enough food for these marginalized farmers to eat can come only from exports. Hence these farmers (as those in Honduras) have responded fairly quickly (with help from the U.S. government) to regional markets, producing such items as snow peas, broccoli, and raspberries. Because agriculture is as profoundly ecological as it is economic, production decisions have local biological effects. These are often environmentally destructive, but the farmers can seldom make changes to avoid such environmental damage without losing the sources of their income. No satisfactory mechanism is in place to change or overrule the market influence so that the local farming practices can be corrected. The necessary feedback loops of economy and policy are missing and need to be deliberately created through policy. Without these loops, we get biological feedbacks of an unpleasant kind—for instance, parasites on raspberries at the consumer end and land degradation and hundreds of cases of pesticide poisoning among Guatemalan farmers every year.

The existing institutional mechanisms for trade in foods were designed to protect North American consumers, without regard for any consequences to the health and well-being of Guatemalans. For instance, the initial governmental response in Canada and the United States to *Cyclospora* contamination of raspberries in the late 1990s was to block Guatemalan raspberry imports. Since this occurred only after the imports seemed to be giving California growers some stiff competition, it is no wonder that one Guatemalan farmer informed me that talking about raspberries was like talking about religion, by which he meant that it had to do with emotions, perceptions, and beliefs manipulated for competitive advantage and not with health at all.

The second response to the contamination of raspberries was to force a few selected producers to institute new hazard control methods, hazards being defined as those that affect North Americans. One recommendation, for instance, was for the farmers to use potable water as a vehicle for spraying pesticides. That is, pesticide toxicity, environmental damage, and lack of clean drinking water are not relevant hazards; the only relevant hazard is the possibility of parasitic infection in North American consumers.

An ecologically and socially sustainable solution to any foodborne disease problem must incorporate the goals of all the major players. This means that the farmers' legitimate need for a livelihood must be addressed systemically, without allowing

the desires of urban consumers to be the primary driving force. The latter results in a global slash-and-burn kind of "sustainability," where wealthy urban consumers satisfy their wants by selectively using up (destroying) local communities and ecosystems around the world. This is a kind of pasture rotation writ large, sustaining the food supply for North Americans even as it destroys the livelihoods of others.

A better approach would include working with the rural Guatemalan agricultural communities to help them find appropriate ecologically and socioeconomically adaptive solutions to foodborne disease problems, which might include better watershed management, education of farm workers, and cooperative growing arrangements. But that would require an acknowledgment that foodborne diseases are as much reflections of political and economic arrangements as they are of technology—an acknowledgment North Americans are loath to make. So, we hear different messages and construct different stories. To address this conundrum, I propose we sit down and listen to each other, and construct a bigger story that has explanatory value for all of us. Storytelling circles and group therapy may be more appropriate models for resolving food safety problems than HACCP and farm-to-fork technologies.

Safe eating, like safe sex, has had a connotation of boredom. But it need not be so. If we reframe the problem, we may see it as an opportunity: to figure out how to prevent bacteria and toxins from sickening our bodies without sabotaging the delicate and intimate relationship between culture and culinary habits. Can it be done? I think so. I would say that the necessary components of any sustainable response to foodborne diseases are a sound understanding of social-ecological interactions across scales, good peripheral vision, and global solidarity.

In coming to grips with the complexity of real life in which foodborne diseases are embedded, we all simplify our approach in some way. Those who simplify the world into a linear, industrial, experimental model tend to hold a simple view of causation (do this and that results) and gravitate toward a series of solutions based on a series of actions along a chain. This is the HACCP approach.

Once the chain is described, one can identify critical points that can be controlled at the farm, by processors, by retailers, and by consumers.

In this scheme of things, consumers are offered a shopping list of rules to protect ourselves. Keep hot things hot (to prevent the bacteria from multiplying) and cold things, like cream pies and potato salad, cold (for the same reason). When you cool things down, do it quickly. This means that the potato salad or the stew should be put in smaller, shallower pots before putting it in the refrigerator; otherwise the outside will cool down while the inside is still incubating the bacteria. Thoroughly scrub the cutting board, counter, and knives after you put the turkey in the oven. Wash your hands after handling raw food. Peel, boil, cook, scrub. Do not eat raw minced meats or milk products. At least singe the bacteria off the outside of your steak.

At its best, this ideology can promote healthy eating without attacking traditional culinary arts. Fermenting walrus meat is supposed to be buried underground, where it is cooler, not hung out in the sun. Perhaps some fermentable carbohydrate can be added to speed up the pH drop. Rice can be cooked in smaller quantities, chilled during storage, and thoroughly reheated before serving. Noodles don't have to be stored at room temperature, eggs don't have to be dirty, and fish can be properly cleaned as soon as they are caught.

Even for chemicals, we are given commandments. Eat less fat. Peel or scrub fruits and vegetables. Avoid foods in which the government reports have identified residues. This way of thinking, however, is not very good at coping with multiple, competing pressures in a complex web of interactions. Washing spinach in the kitchen is useless if it was contaminated by *E. coli* on the farm as a result of economic market forces that "demanded" low-priced, "naturally produced," "fresh" food. I put all those words in quotation marks because they are all disputable terms.

Linear causal systems also tend to give critical points in the system equal weight. If meat from a poultry production unit (I hesitate to call it a farm) is highly contaminated with *Salmonella,* it may negate the simple precautions that consumers take in their homes. One response to this is what I would call the bulldozer solution: massive regulation and control. Send everyone to the supermarket to buy canned, packaged, or irradiated food and ask them to put away childish barbecues and eat well-cooked chickenlike meat and hamburgers at fast food restaurants. This way of thinking can transform a legitimate public health concern about the safety of raw milk into a Monty Python–esque police raid on a farm to empty the milk tank of a farmer who was selling unpasteurized milk to consenting adults, as happened in Ontario in 2006.

The application of linear causal thinking in a complex world creates a dozen new problems for everyone involved. Farmers lower *Salmonella* contamination at the farm through stringent all-in, all-out, essentially quarantined specific-pathogen-free flocks. Food processors get rid of the remainder at the plant through irradiation and chemicals. Mass production (economies of scale), together with subsidized fossil fuel costs, keeps the prices down for consumers. In the meantime, the genetic base of farm animal populations is homogenized and narrowed, creating large populations of animals susceptible to pandemic diseases ranging from *Salmonella* to avian influenza. Economic power has been centralized in the agrifood industry, and society is committed to energy inefficiency and increased vulnerability. The overall system promotes global warming, which is already associated with increasing the rates of foodborne illnesses everywhere.

A more realistic, scientifically based approach acknowledges that foodborne diseases are affected by climate change, environmental resilience, the distance the food travels, personal eating habits, social and economic inequities, power relations in society, culture, and microbial ecology. Diarrhea and vomiting cannot easily be balanced against the risks of cancer, however murky the data, and the pests and diseases that plague modern agriculture are not adequate justification for the use of those chemicals; an increase in infectious foodborne diseases may be nature's rallying cry for a complete restructuring of our food-producing system, rather than a call for more pills.

Each of us has some power and responsibility to eat safely. I do not want to worry about what might be in my food, however. I don't mind some danger. I do mind unnecessary risks. We need to address not only personal hygiene but also questions of why these bacteria, parasites, and chemicals are floating around in our food ecology at all. Is it because crop insurance companies demand that pesticides and antibacterial drugs be used? Is it that some industrialists tell us we will all starve if we don't keep doing things the way we are? Is it because we are obsessed with personal health, and the world (our children, other species, poor people everywhere) be damned?

Instead of starting with the pieces and building a food chain, I think it's useful to imagine the whole, to integrate our concepts and our actions internally and with each other. Several concepts from the scholarly work on complexity theory are helpful here: feedback loops, holonocracy, resilience, and post-normal science. It sounds like rocket science, but it's not. It is a new kind of common sense. Bear with me.

Every outcome is the cause of something else, which, through a series of links over time and space, affect a wide range of outcomes, including, often, what you started with. This is a feedback loop, and this book is full of examples. Promotion of efficiency in meat processing to solve economic and environmental problems led to recycling unused meat, which led to an epidemic of BSE and massive waste in the cattle industry. Promotion of food irradiation as a food safety technology (to prevent the sale of contaminated meat) encourages economies of scale (because of the costs of the irradiators) and a globalization of markets (to support the increased output from the food processor). Economies of scale for livestock are associated with crowding large groups of animals, which leads to higher rates of bacterial shedding from the animals and thus higher rates of meat contamination. The globalization of trade ensures that the contaminated products are more widely circulated. Furthermore, this now centralized food system is based on a high rate of fossil fuel input, which changes the climate, resulting in more extreme weather events. The existing large-scale system is very poor at adapting to the sudden changes which are, in many respects, of its own making. How you solve the problem of a foodborne disease will affect other social, ecological, and health problems—if not now, then a few years down the road.

Holonocracy is a bit more complicated. I think of it this way: I am an individual, with my own internal psychological and biophysical rules that keep me going; I am also a part of a family, which has its own internal rules and sets of interactions; my family is part of several larger communities, each of which has its own internal rules and interactions. I can imagine a similar nested hierarchy about myself using ecological units. In fact, for any phenomenon, I can create many such nested hierarchies. Each of the units in the hierarchy is both a whole and a part. The philosopher of science Arthur Koestler christened these units holons; the nested hierarchies have gone by various names. I prefer that proposed by environmental scientist Henry Regier—holonocracy—because it suggests an alternative to autocracy and conventional democracy.

In the context of the agrifood system, that means I need to think of myself as both an individual and a part. My eating habits are related to my history and culture and the society in which I live; by the same token changes in large cultures and ecosystems (such as the price of oil, the climate, or religious ideologies) can determine whether or not individuals get sick. Any sustainable food safety system needs to pay attention to feedback loops across scales.

Resilience is the ability of a system to keep self-organizing and functioning even as it deals with major stresses and catastrophes. We all want the agrifood system to keep providing us with food, fiber, safe water, and (for many) employment. Resilience implies that these functions can still be performed if climates change, prices drop, oil dries up, and populations migrate.

Finally, postnormal science is a way of thinking about and doing science developed by philosophers of science Silvio Funtowicz and Jerry Ravetz. When scientists and the societies in which they live are faced with situations in which the facts are in dispute, there are ethical arguments and conflicts over what constitutes legitimate knowledge and in which there is some urgency to make policy and management decisions. In these kinds of situations (which those who work on environmental and public health issues will recognize), Funtowicz and Ravetz say that nothing "can be managed in a convenient isolation; issues are mutually implicated; problems extend across many scale levels of space and time; and uncertainties and value-loadings of all sorts and all degrees of severity affect data and theories alike."

Without going into a deep discussion here, they make the point that scientists need to expand their peer group to include a wide range of citizens who are affected by the system, people with different kinds of knowledge and power, to work toward a common understanding of what is going on and what we can do about it. This kind of postnormal science, which is different from what one might call postmodern science, where different views of the world merely compete, poses far more challenges than ordinary science and ordinary social action. It requires an openness to different ideas, ways of dealing with issues of gender and political and economic power, and new ways of assessing the quality of the information we are using.

Is this pie-in-the sky? It is not. I have seen it work, but it requires a citizenry that is biologically knowledgeable and socially engaged. Which is one reason I have written this book, as my way of contributing to the discussion.

We do not yet know the appropriate size or the degree of variability required for an agricultural and food system that might last a million years, which is the average life expectancy of a mammalian species, or a hundred million years, which is how long the dinosaurs lasted. What is clear is that if we do not begin to think about these things now, we may not have another chance.

Taking this complexness and sorting through it in my head, I tend to come back to some version of health—not so much my personal health, although that's important to me, but the health of the planet. In human and animal health, we do not measure success purely by longevity. We measure the ability to do what we desire, resilience, and coping skills, and hope that longevity follows. In social-ecological systems, the dimensions of health include the integrity of the biophysical environment, socioeconomic resilience, and the health and well-being of the people who produce and consume the bounty of agricultural lands. This kind of full resource accounting takes us far beyond both the narrow financial bookkeeping of neoconservative economists and the endless toxin identification espoused by some environmental groups. It takes our concerns with individual health seriously but puts them in an appropriate larger context.

We might find ourselves asking odd questions. There have been suggestions in the scientific literature that people who have had parasites as children are less likely to suffer some kinds of allergic symptoms, including, perhaps, asthma. There is also evidence that, for some bacteria, exposure in childhood can result in resistance (although it can also result in disease and death). I suggest further that the ability to respond to outbreaks would soon atrophy in a society that had no foodborne disease, and that a healthy person is someone who can recover from bouts of illness, rather than someone who never gets sick. When I am reasoning this way, I ask, "How much foodborne disease is actually a good amount?"

Considering the way foodborne diseases have moved around the world, I am also led to ask whether the microbes that cause Montezuma's revenge or Casablanca crud are just doing their job. Much disease occurs because the things we take for granted, such as clean water and adequate sewage disposal, are not available in Mexico City and Casablanca. By creating food safety programs in North America or Europe that focus only on protecting consumers, rather than spending similar sums of money in developing countries to help them create well-managed water and sewer systems and more sustainable farming practices, we put the entire system at risk. We live in one interacting globe. When tourists go south and suffer the natural consequences of eating contaminated food or drinking contaminated water, they are reaping the consequences of systemic inequities embedded in agrifood systems that were designed, supposedly, to protect them. Furthermore, because of those inequities, the diseases are not waiting for tourists to come to them; they are traveling north in foods grown in those contaminated environments.

We cannot avoid government regulation and public vigilance, but they will not solve all our problems. We cannot legislate everything. The decisions we make about how to provide safe food for ourselves cannot be left to government, which will succumb to the financially numbing pressure of financially powerful interest groups. Nor can it be left to scientists, whose pieces of information are necessary but not sufficient. But individuals cannot go it alone either. For one thing, most of us do not want to spend all our waking hours thinking about food. For another, the solutions to our problems—not just those related to food but the whole connected mess we live in—will by their nature require collective action.

One of my frustrations in talking about food to my fellow urbanites is that they do not understand the dimensions and seriousness of the problems we are facing. Maybe we need to put into place laws and tax structures to encourage sophisticated, small-scale, diversified farming within the city limits. Every housing estate should encompass at least one active food-producing farm and an abattoir. If there is a conflict between urban uses or agriculture, farming should automatically be given precedence; farms should be pushing back, invading the city, and not vice versa. We can live without car factories and textile mills; we cannot live without food. With food production right under their noses, urbanites might actually come to understand what the real issues are and make informed choices.

I am not talking about going back to some good old days. I am talking about relaxing our dietary obsessions, whether they be for beef, broccoli, chicken, or cabbage. We need to be less fanatical in our attachment to the industrialization of agriculture, supported by huge subsidies of energy and nutrients, and less addicted to technological and chemical control. We need to go beyond good bookkeeping and sloppy biology to a much more refined and sophisticated cultural arrangement, one that accounts intelligently for our true place in nature. What does this mean? How can this happen? Can an individual make a difference? Where everything seems to be connected to everything else, what hope is there for an individual to make a difference? The systemic connections in the real world between environmental sustainability, public health, economic efficiency, cultural preferences, and so on can be seen as an opportunity for hope, rather than despair. An accumulation of small actions can bring the whole system to a kind of tipping point, resulting in a cascade of changes (most of which, we hope, are good). When talking to schoolchildren I use the example of red blood cells. If you lose one cell, does it bother you? Two? Seven? One hundred? A quart full? And yet, at some point, a person has bled to death. Every cell in some way makes a difference, and a transfusion of thousands of individual red blood cells at a key moment can save a life, and result in positive changes across a wide range of outcomes.

During my stay in Guatemala, I went with a small group of students to visit a coffee *finca* and processing plant in the central highlands. The head coffee taster and quality-control specialist talked to us about the color variations in raw and roasted beans and about hundreds of subtle flavors that could be detected in different coffees. He showed us how to slurp, gargle, and spit. We learned about the highest grades of beans, those that produce the richest flavors, which grow on coffee bushes that require shade trees, and thus need a complex and relatively stable ecosystem to thrive.

He explained to us that Americans, who consume huge amounts of coffee every year, do not generally care about quality. Of all the major coffee-importing countries, he said that the U.S. has the lowest official quality standards; Canada has slightly higher, and Europe has the highest. One small consequence of this, according to our taster-guide, was that one of the chief tasters for a major U.S. company smokes cigarettes, apparently without it interfering with his job. He himself does not smoke, drink alcohol, eat spicy foods—or even drink coffee!—in order to keep his senses fresh and clean. There are more serious consequences than mediocre coffee, however, to having generally low standards. Varieties of coffee that do not require shade are also more productive. If the goal is a large amount of cheap coffee, non-shade coffee appears to be more *efficient*. Hence there are strong economic incentives to cut down all the trees, and, with a fair amount of help from high doses of pesticides and fertilizers, grow lots of low-grade coffee. In one study in Central America, this resulted in the loss not only of all the trees, but also of 128 species of beetle, 103 species of wasps, and 17 species of foraging ants. While ants may not qualify as charismatic mega-fauna (like elephants or pandas), there is evidence that they can protect coffee plants against some major insect plagues. But of course we have more pesticides for that.

Guatemala, furthermore, has 734 known species of orchids, 738 species of birds, 124 species of bromeliads, and 519 species of mosses, all of which require trees or at least shade to thrive. Obsessed with a single goal—efficient production of large quantities—we ignore others—quality, environmental integrity, workers' livelihoods—which translates into Central American deforestation, loss of heartbreakingly great beauty and diversity, increased use of various pesti-, fungi-, etcetera-cides (that is, chemicals that kill things), and increased ecological fragility.

Market-price efficiency is not *wrong* as a goal. However, pursued in its own right, without reference to social and ecological context, rather than as one component of a more complex goal such as a sustainable, healthy planet, it has become a life-destroying obsession. It makes sense to adopt multiple criteria for coffee production: justice and fair prices for farmers; safeguarding the integrity of ecosystems. By doing so, we may reduce efficiency, but we also endorse a sustainable and healthy planet. These criteria should be applied to all products, not just coffee. What can a person do? Buy local, if you can. Buy organic as much as possible, but, as I suggested in chapter 9, prefer local nonorganic to trucked-in organic. Buy fair trade. Pay attention at the grocery store. Ask the manager where the food comes from. The cumulative impact of small individual decisions can be enormous.

Some wonderful meals are worth the risks they entail, and I have been known to rationalize the purchase of an expensive green pepper grown no doubt under exploitive conditions far outside my own bioregion, just so I can make a proper sweet-and-sour dish. I kept my wooden cutting board when scientists said plastic was safer and was delighted when they changed their minds. But that's beside the point. I wasn't using a wooden cutting board because it was safer; I was using it because, whatever its safety record, I liked the feel of it.

But I do clean the counter after preparing chicken. Other risks, especially those that go beyond my personal culinary tastes and put at risk the innocent (children) or the biotic environment in which we all live are unacceptable and require vigorous political action (and yes, that might include my green pepper, depending on its origin). We need efficiency, substitution of benign products for hazardous ones, *and* restructuring of our social and agricultural arrangements. The world is too complex for anything less than that. I hope that this book will help people to make intelligent choices and provide them with at least some of the information needed to select among the choices available to us.

In *The Parable of the Beast,* John Bleibtreu has written about the possible biological sources of our mythologies and rituals. After discussions about how insects establish their sense of self, community, and "otherness" through the sharing of various chemicals, he goes on to speculate about how Christian communion fits into this larger natural pattern. In a very real, genetic sense, we have learned from the ants. Jesus came eating and drinking and was called a glutton and a drinker, a friend of tax-gatherers and sinners, and his followers instituted a meal, the communion, a continuation of the Jewish Passover meal, as their most intimate and powerful affirmation of community.

In almost every culture, we accord central importance to the act of eating together, of letting go and trusting that what our fellow human beings have grown and prepared for us is safe and nourishing. Eating together is an act of friendship, romance, and family life. In evolutionary terms, it is an embodiment of a vital truth, the survival benefits of sharing a meal, the trust that this entails for everyone involved, and the necessity of that group trust for species survival. Eating a meal is a microcosm of our planetary life, of the need for us all to go out on a limb for each other if we are to survive.

It is also a reminder that, through our food, within us and around us, millions of microscopic beings are speaking, whispering to us of our mortality, of the membership dues each of us must pay for being party to this green and wondrous celebration. In my opinion, the dues are well worth paying. Wash your hands. Talk with your friends. Question authority. Contribute to the debate. Examine the evidence. Change your mind. Eat on.

CHICKEN SOUP FOR THE BODY

Mennonite Comfort for a Fall Day in New Suburbia

Over the back fence, call to the neighbors
by their pool. Invite them for supper.
Using a long pole with a hook on the end
snatch a chicken by the leg.
Drag her squawking through the dust.
Grasp both legs firmly.
Lay the neck firmly across the top of the stump.
Raise the ax slowly. Say a prayer.
With your eyes open, swing hard and true.
Let the body have one last romp around the yard
little red fountains leaping from the neck-stump.
Laugh outrageously with the kids.
Plunge the exhausted body into a tub of hot water.
Sit in the shade of the giant black walnut tree,
plucking out the feathers, singing old hymns.
The prickly pin feathers are the most difficult.
Let the kids work at those. They have small fingers.
As a reward for helping, the kids can play
with the chicken feet;
they can pull the tendons from inside shirt-sleeves,
screaming with delight as they yank
witch's claws open and shut at the neighbors.
Rinse off the plucked bird. Cut carefully
at the base of the neck. Tie off the esophagus.
Slit open the abdomen.
Play with the intestines, slipping them
through your fingers like fat worms.
Tie off the rectum. Cut around it.
Reach deeply up into the abdominal cavity.
Scoop out everything in one big slippery heap,

trimming away attachments as necessary.
Set aside the heart, liver, and the gizzard.
In Indonesia, they rinse out the intestines
and make a special soup from them,
but most Canadians do not find this comforting,
so just toss the remaining offal into the garbage.
Rinse out the cavity.
Place the empty body into a pot
with the neck, liver, heart, and gizzard.
Add just enough water so the body floats.
Sprinkle a teaspoon of salt into your palm
and brush it into the pot with your other hand.
After about forty minutes, add the dumplings
(see separate recipe).
Dollop the dough like puffy pillows
on the breasts, the wings, the thighs.
Ten minutes covered.
Ten minutes uncovered.
Teach the neighbours how to sing the doxology
in four-part harmony.
Spoon the chicken and dumplings on to large white plates.
Serve with fresh peas.
Save the heart and liver for yourself
as a treat. High in iron, you know.
Let the dog chew on the gizzard.
Dad usually likes the neck.
At dusk, after the guests have gone home, don't forget
to go out to feed the chickens.

FURTHER READING

For those of you who are interested in pursuing some of the subjects raised in this book from a more technical standpoint, the following will give you a start.

Cliver, D.O., ed. 2002. *Foodborne Diseases*, 2nd ed. Toronto: Academic Press.

Funtowicz, S.O., and J.R. Ravetz. 1990. *Uncertainty and Quality in Science for Policy*. Dordrecht: Kluwer.

———. 1991. Three Types of Risk Assessment and the Emergence of Post-normal Science. In D. Golding and S. Krimsky (eds.) *Social Theories of Risk*. New York: Greenwood.

———90. 1993. Science for the Post-normal Age. *Futures* 25(7): 739–755.Heymann, D. 2004. *Control of Communicable Diseases Manual*, 18th ed. Washington: American Public Health Association.

Hui, Y., ed. 1994. *Foodborne Disease Handbook. Vol. 1: Diseases Caused by Bacteria Vol. 2: Diseases Caused by Viruses, Parasites and Fungi Vol. 3: Diseases Caused by Hazardous Substances*. New York: M. Dekker.

International Association of Milk, Food, and Environmental Sanitarians. Committee on Communicable Diseases Affecting Man. 1999. *Procedures to Investigate Foodborne Illness*, 5th edition (revised 2007). Des Moines, IA: Interna-

tional Association of Milk, Food, and Environmental
Sanitarians, Inc.

Mortimore, S., and C.A. Wallace. 1998. HACCP: *A Practical
Approach,* 2nd ed. New York: Springer.

Riemann, H., and F. Bryan. 1979. *Foodborne Infections and
Intoxications.* Toronto: Academic Press.

Winter, C.K., J.N. Seiber, and C.F. Nuckton, eds. 1990.
Chemicals in the Human Food Chain. New York: Van
Nostrand Reinhold.

JOURNALS

The *Journal of Food Protection* is the major reference journal
in this subject area. Some of the other journals which report on
foodborne illnesses are *Emerging Infectious Diseases, EcoHealth,
The American Journal of Public Health, The Canadian Journal
of Public Health, The New England Journal of Medicine, Epidemiology and Infection,* and *The Lancet.* For chemical residues,
The Journal of the Association of Official Analytical Chemists
contains articles on both methodology and national survey
results. Quite frankly, I don't think any of us who do research
could survive without the scholarly bulletin board and international information exchange PubMed.

The following government reports include foodborne
diseases:

Public Health & Epidemiology Report Ontario (PHERO),
formerly Ontario Disease Surveillance Report (ODSR).
This can be ordered from the Public Health Branch of the
Ontario Ministry of Health and Long-Term Care.

Canadian Disease Weekly Review (CDWR), put out by the
Public Health Agency of Canada.

Morbidity and Mortality Weekly Report (MMWR), U.S. Department of Health and Human Services, Centers for Disease
Control and Prevention, Atlanta.

GENERAL READING

Berton Roueche's *Annals of Epidemiology* (Boston: Little, Brown, 1967) and *The Medical Detectives* Vol. ii (New York : E.P. Dutton, 1984) have some good whodunits in them, and *The Ballad of Typhoid Mary* (New York: Ballantine, 1985) by J.F. Federspiel is a classic. To these I would add Robert Desowitz's *New Guinea Tapeworms and Jewish Grandmothers: Tales of Parasites and People* (New York: Avon Books, 1981).

Eric Schlosser's book on the American agrifood system, *Fast Food Nation* (Boston: Houghton Mifflin, 2001), should be read by everyone who eats. He is an excellent and observant reporter.

A good general book on food and the allure, obsessions, mythology, perils, and taboos surrounding it is Margaret Visser's *Much Depends on Dinner* (Toronto: McClelland & Stewart, 1986).

ACKNOWLEDGMENTS

T HIS IS THE kind of book for which the acknowledgments could be as long as the book itself. Thanks to NC Press for taking a chance on me and publishing the first edition. Thanks to my agent, Carolyn Swayze, and to Rob Sanders at Greystone Books for giving the book a second life. Special thanks to Elizabeth and Stan Litch for the use of their log cabin on the escarpment. It is a most wonderful writing space. Thanks to the students of Epidemiology of Foodborne Diseases at the University of Guelph, who have tolerated my explorations of this subject matter since 1987 and have questioned me, challenged me, kept me interested, and educated me with their creative essays and dissemination projects. Dr. Linda Harris, now at the University of Davis in California, is a formidable (and friendly!) food microbiologist. Linda co-taught this course with me for several years and managed to keep me almost microbiologically correct. In recent years, as the size of the class exploded, I could not have survived without my teaching assistants. Drs. Dominique Charron (now director of EcoHealth Programs at the International

Development Research Centre), Sandy Lefebvre, and Andria Jones deserve special mention. Andria taught the course when I was on a sabbatical semester, helped me fill in the details on my "vision stuff," and co-authored a paper with me on creative teaching methods.

Dr. Shannon Majowicz co-taught a graduate course on special topics in public health with me, and Dominique Charron co-taught a course with me on systems approaches to ecology and health. Thanks to both the co-instructors and the students; I think I learned as much as I taught in both courses.

The work of some of the recent graduate students I have collaborated with has contributed to this new edition and given me new insights into the challenges facing society in dealing with foodborne and waterborne illnesses. In particular, the work of Karen Morrison on ciguatera, Kate Thomas on extreme rainfall and waterborne disease outbreaks, and Andria Jones on why people drink bottled water come to mind.

When I first started teaching the course, I could read all the literature and summarize it in my lectures. Twenty years later, this was impossible, as the scholarly literature on foodborne illnesses has exploded. So I need to thank all my colleagues who have stepped into the breach and given guest lectures when I felt overwhelmed.

This book is based on a lot of research, mine and others, mostly since the 1980s. Much of what appears here is based on extensive searches in the peer-reviewed literature, as well as some previous scholarly publications of my own. Some of my ideas on foodborne illnesses were partly developed (half baked?) in these papers, including: "One ecosystem, one food system: the social and ecological context of food safety strategies," in the *Journal of Agricultural and Environmental Ethics* (1991, 4:49–59), which itself was a reworking of an invited talk I gave at the Globe '90 conference in Vancouver, British Columbia; and in an invited editorial in the *Canadian Journal of Public Health* (July/August 1991) with a title the same as that of this book. The chapter on radionuclides in food is largely based on my article in the *Canadian Veterinary Journal* (1990, 31:361–366) entitled "Food safety in a nuclear crisis: the role of the veterinarian," which itself was based on an invited talk I gave at a convention of the Canadian Veterinary Medical Association. "Grandma's Revenge" started as a talk I gave at a convention of the Canadian Public Health Association in 1990.

For the chapters on chemicals, I drew heavily on a report prepared in 1991 by Dr. Scott McEwen and me for the Ontario Ministry of Agriculture and Food entitled *Human Health Risks from Chemical Contaminants in Foods of Animal Origin,* which was published as a special edition of *Veterinary Public Health* (August 1994, 20:161–247). I also drew on two scholarly papers on developing a systemic understanding of, and hence systemic responses to, foodborne illnesses: "A new conceptual base for food and agricultural policy: the emerging model of links between agriculture, food, health, environment and society," which I co-wrote with Tim Lang and which appeared in *Global Change and Human Health* (2001, 1(2):116–130); and "An Agroecosystem perspective on foodborne illness," which was published in *Ecosystem Health* (1996, 2:177–185).

INDEX